Too Old to Ultra?

When a marathon is just not enough.
If an older athlete, like me, can still log
the long miles - maybe you can too.

Stephen Morley

ISBN: 9781073525737

Photographs by. A.B. Johnson

Welcome to my book, Too Old to Ultra. It's something of a follow up to my previous book, Running with a Wounded Heart. That book tells the story of how I took up running in later life, became obsessed with racing as a senior athlete and during my 50s, while competing, ultimately had a heart attack, the book talks about my recovery and how I went on to register a personal best marathon time in my sixties. Since completing that book in 2013, I discovered the wonderful world of Ultrarunning. There are differing opinions on what constitutes an Ultra. I've always heard that ultra is any race longer than 32 miles. It sounds big-headed to say that I'd become bored with running marathons, however, I had completed in quite a few and while I still had a few big city marathons on my bucket list, I was increasingly drawn to the longer distances.

This book is the story of my love affair with Ultras, what they are and where to find them. I've also written about some of the most memorable ultra-races and the men and women who run them. The book is called Too Old to Ultra and as a senior runner myself, I'm interested in what it takes for the more mature runner to train and compete in races longer than the standard marathon distance. As well as the physical impact, I examine the mental resolve needed to be on your feet for many hours and explore the medical implications for older runners. Throughout the book, I also invite you to share in one or two ultra-adventures including my own disastrous first attempt.

I hope that you enjoy the book.

Disclaimer

Any advice and suggestions contained in this book are based on research and personal experience. I am not a professional athlete, athletics coach, or doctor. If you are an older person taking up running or any physical activity for the first time you should consult your doctor and get their ok before you begin. In my opinion, you shouldn't attempt an ultra until you have completed at least a few marathons first.

Dedication

I'd like to dedicate this book to my best friend and running buddy, Quang Le. Le has been with me on my running journey since the beginning. I've lost count of the races we have competed in, not to mention the, probably, thousands of miles we have covered together in training. He is the perfect running partner and seems to know instinctively when I've had enough and need to walk and when I'm just feeling lazy and need a bit of a kick. We had run several marathons together,

However, up until now I've yet to persuade him to do an ultra with me. He always tells me that I'm crazy – he is probably right.

Table of Contents.

Contributors

About the Author

Bonus content
Exerts from a Podcast

Thank you and final thoughts

Preface

Peddars Way Ultra Marathon Saturday 31st January 2015.

The conditions were appalling and only a last-minute decision was made to go ahead with the race.

I think a lot of the faster runners wanted to get finished before dark and before the really bad weather closed in and temperatures dropped any lower.

As usual, I went off too quickly and my heart rate was a bit high. However, I soon settled into the run and reached the first checkpoint at 13 miles without too much trouble. Having said that, it was very wet and muddy underfoot. Snow and sleet had been falling heavily, pretty much from the start.

Despite the conditions, I was setting a reasonable pace. The next checkpoint was at 26.5 miles, approx. half distance at a place called Castle Acre.

Conditions got progressively worse and at about 17 miles I found myself running into a blizzard. The sleet was burning my eyes and face. At about 18 miles I found myself running along the top of an embankment. There were large sections of the path that were waterlogged, very muddy, with large frozen puddles. Visibility was poor, my eyes were watering and in trying to avoid one of the larger puddles I ran to the side and lost my footing in the mud. As I slipped my foot hit a tree root and I went over. Unfortunately, because I was on the edge of the embankment there was nowhere for me to go but down and so I fell headlong into a drainage ditch.

Chapter 1.   What is an Ultra

As I mentioned in my introduction, my definition of an Ultra is any race over 32 miles. However, its officially called an Ultra Marathon. With that in mind, the listing in Wikipedia gives the following definition, *"An ultramarathon, also called ultra-distance or ultra-running, is any footrace longer than the traditional marathon length of 42.195 kilometers"*.   So, it's safe to say that an ultramarathon is any race extending beyond the standard marathon running distance of 42 kilometers, 195 meters (26 miles, 385 yards). Ultra-races typically begin at 50 kilometers and can extend to enormous distances.

Since the sport is becoming increasingly popular, you will find so-called beginner ultras starting from around 32 miles right up to mega ultras like the Badwater Ultramarathon and the Marathon des Sables. Both vie for the title *"The Toughest Footrace on Earth"*. Both races are certainly the stuff of legends.

New long-distance events are being introduced all the time but a candidate for the World's longest ultramarathon is the aptly named *"The Ultimate Ultra"*, officially called the annual Sri Chinmoy 1300-Miler (2092 kilometers). This formidable race is held every year in New York, USA. There is also the Trans America Footrace. Competitors race from Los Angeles to New York over 64 consecutive days, covering a phenomenal distance of 3,000 miles.

So, since this book is called *"Too old to ultra,"* let's make our point early and mention that, In 2014, William Sichel duly completed Trans America in 50 days, 15 hours, 6 minutes and 4 seconds becoming the first person from Britain to complete the event inside the 52-day time limit. He was also the first person aged over 60 to finish the race since it started in 1997. Just for good measure, it's worth saying that he accomplished these achievements despite having previously had cancer.

But back to the races themselves. As you can see, in terms of distance, there is no limit to what qualifies as an ultra.

Many runners graduate to ultrarunning after competing in marathons and are looking for greater challenges.

Interestingly, ultramarathon racing has been around longer than the *marathon (which originated with the first modern Olympics in 1896)* but it's only relatively recently that the sport has been recognized by the International Amateur Athletic Federation (IAAF). In 1991, the IAAF extended official recognition to the 100-kilometer event. Since that time the 100-kilometer event has replaced the marathon as the longest running distance recognized by the world athletics governing body. The annual International Association of Ultrarunners (IAU) 100-Kilometer World Challenge is now held each year by the IAU under the patronage of the IAAF.

Ultramarathons can be run on any surface, roads, forest, mountain trails and rocky tracks. They can be run from your start at point A to your finish (usually many, many miles later) at point B.

The famous Comrades Marathon in South Africa is an example of a point to point race where runners run between Durban and Pietermaritzburg.

Interestingly each year the Comrades changes around its start and finish, one-year competitors, run from Durban to Pietermaritzburg and the following year from Pietermaritzburg to Durban.

The Comrades is on my bucket list.

One of the biggest differences between a standard marathon and an ultra-marathon, apart from the longer distances involved, is that it's quite normal to take walking breaks, stop to eat and drink and even sit or lay down for rest breaks. For the longer multi-day events competitors will have sleep/rest breaks at the end of each day's *"run"* The runners don't incur any penalties by taking these breaks, except for the time or distance a runner loses from their overall performance. In truth, unlike running a marathon, when taking part in an ultra-event, time is not such a big consideration. I'm not talking about the elite men and women of the sport here. They are a breed apart.

I well remember first reading about Scott Jurek. I had naively compared an average marathon pace to an ultramarathon.

I had assumed that, running so much longer would equate to a much slower pace. Then I came across this peice from an American running magazine

Reporter: *I guess as an ultramarathon runner, completing a marathon is just a short training run, right?*

Scott Jurek: *Well, I don't want to say it's just like brushing my teeth, but to run around in 3hr 30min ... I mean, I want to respect the distance, but it feels comfortable. Almost like a warm-up.*

As far as yours truly is concerned, I am focused on surviving and getting to the finish line. That is my primary objective.

If I can stay on the right side of any race organizer's mandatory cut off times, my actual finishing time is usually the last thing on my mind.

Chapter 2.   How far

"Peddars" or The Peddars Way Ultra Marathon, to give it its full title, runs from the Suffolk border to the North Norfolk Coast. At approx. 48 miles it falls into the *"beginner"* category as far as ultra runs are concerned. On the Peddars Way website, the route is described as very runnable, even in the winter and navigation is said to be easy. Please make a note of that last statement. I found myself repeating these words, many, many times, through gritted teeth and snow stung eyes while struggling to keep my feet (very runnable) and find my way (navigation easy) in a blizzard. But more of that later.

To enter the race, you must be aged 21 years or over on the date of the race. You must have completed a run of at least 26.2 in the last 12 months and have experience of running off-road.

I can't remember how I first heard about Peddars. It's possible that I read about the race in one of my many running magazines. However, I do remember people's reaction when I first mentioned my intention to take it on.

You want to run how far? That was the reaction I got from Stuart, the manager of the Inspire Fitness gym at the time. Stuart was a fit guy and had taken part in several *"Tough Mudder"* races.

The Tough Mudder is a series of hardcore 10-12-mile obstacle races - mud run events designed by British Special Forces to challenge the toughest of the tough. So, he was no stranger to the concept of taking on a challenge.

However, I can still remember him asking me how far the Peddars race was. ***"48 miles? That's a bloody long way to run Steve"***.

I was confident that I could cover 48 miles. Notice I said covered and not run. Most people who take on an ultra, do so knowing that they will need to walk for at least part of the distance. Having said that I'm amazed at the number of non-runners, who assume that these longer distance races are done at the same speed as say, your average marathon...only for an extra 86.9 miles.

For the elite ultrarunners that is often true. Since I didn't and don't consider myself in that league, running the whole way wasn't in my plans.

As things turned out, I didn't get to find out if I could have completed that distance. I did, however, have a challenge of a very different type to overcome.

Chapter 3.   Very runnable

So, there I was laying on my back in a drainage ditch. I would like to tell you all that I fell down a ravine because that would sound more dramatic. If I tell you it was a drainage ditch you will probably laugh at me. It knocked the wind out of me, and I bruised my shoulder, but it was the fact that I twisted my ankle on the tree root that did me in. I climbed out of the ravine, sorry drainage ditch, a little wet and sore but in not too bad a shape. However, when I tried to run, my ankle was quite painful. I tried to run it off, but it wasn't looking good. I was in the middle of nowhere in the teeth of a blizzard and a good eight and a half miles away from the nearest checkpoint.

Well, I did the only thing I could. I started to cry. Not really. We old boys are made of sterner stuff. I walked, hobbled, tried to run a bit and hobbled a bit more. Eventually, I got within a couple of miles of the checkpoint. By now the snow was falling heavily and all the signs were getting covered. It was at this point that I was reminded of the words on the Peddars Way website, *very runnable and easy to navigate, even in the winter.*

Because I had to walk, I was starting to get very cold, particularly my hands and feet. I found a post with an Acorn sign on it, *(distinctive acorn symbols on stiles, gates, and signposts to mark running and walking routes).* but by the time I'd gone 3 miles I realized it must have been for a different route and I'd gone the wrong way. So, I had to backtrack. Yes, yes, Ok, I admit it. I was lost.

The bad weather was closing in and even though it was still the only afternoon, it was starting to get very dark and overcast. I had met another runner, rather comically coming toward me from the opposite direction. He was the first runner, the first person, I had seen in a couple of hours. I wasn't the only one lost. *"I'm heading for Castle Acre,"* I said. *"I saw a sign that said this way"* *"Well I've just been down that way"* he replied, *"and, I saw a sign that said Castle Acre this way."* We both bust out laughing. Having spent several minutes exchanging tales of woe, moaning about the weather, the race organizers, our bad luck and life in general, we decided to knock at a nearby farmhouse and ask for directions.

We had both decided that, whatever happened, we were both calling it quits once we managed to get to the next checkpoint. My new friend had had enough and there was no way I was going to make it to 48 miles, walking with a sore ankle in the snow. Armed with new directions we were soon back on track heading for the checkpoint. Once resigned to calling it a day, I started looking forward to the end of my misery. All the checkpoints have food and hot drinks available. Castle Acre, being the approximate halfway point had race volunteers serving hot soup, an assortment of hot food and blankets ready to welcome cold and weary runners.

I finally got to Castle Acre, having run, walked, and hobbled a total of 32 miles. (It should have been 26.5) and could almost smell the lovely hot soup and warming food. As the checkpoint came into view it appeared to be deserted. A lone table and a race organizers banner, but no volunteers and no soup, hot food or blankets. Just an empty table and snow-covered race banner.

As it turned out, the race organizers had decided that the cut off time should be brought forward so only the faster runners had been allowed to continue. The race organizers were concerned about slower runners getting caught in worsening weather after dark. Because of this, the checkpoint had been taken down, food, hot drinks, and blankets packed away and no volunteers to be seen.

Fortunately, there was a pub close by. I said goodbye to my fellow runner, he had telephoned ahead, and a lift was waiting for him and made my way to the pub hoping to get myself a hot Tea or Coffee. Once inside I quickly found what had happened to the volunteers. They were sitting at a table in the lovely warm pub, enjoying their Sunday lunches. I remember the volunteer in charge picking up his phone and saying

"Hello race control, Castle Acre here. Runner number 689 has just arrived, how many is it now we are still missing?"

I didn't know if to laugh or cry.

The decision to bring the cut-off point forward was a good one though. It wasn't just the slower runners that were suffering. Several guys in the top group of runners abandoned due to hypothermia.

To be fair to the organizers, as I understand it, this particular year was particularly harsh as far as the weather was concerned. Even though the race is run in January, there have been many years when runners have taken part in the cold but bright winter sunshine.

I'm not sure if I would have made the revised cut off point had I not had the fall. But, in the end, it was academic. Still, apart from a sore shoulder and an aching foot, I was none the worse for wear and lived to fight another day.

The day after the race I found myself reading the race reviews on Facebook and the various Ultra-Forums. All the posts had one word in common, *"Brutal"* Apparently over a third of the runners failed to finish. I certainly picked a good one for my first ultra. I was disappointed not to have made it to the finish. Still, it was pointed out to me that since I had run 32 miles, albeit by getting lost, it did qualify as an ultra. So, I had officially run my first ultra, just no T-Shirt, finisher's medal, and no cigar, oh hum.

Close but no cigar!

Despite the crazy weather, the fall, the injuries, and all the adverse weather conditions, strangely, I found the whole adventure exhilarating and wanted some more.

Chapter 4.   How old is too old

My Son-in-law came to collect me and apparently, I didn't look in great shape. I'd only fallen down a ravine, sorry drainage ditch, twisted an ankle and battled 32 miles through a blizzard. I can't think why I wasn't looking my best. In any event, having had a heart attack in 2010, my family were naturally concerned about my health. Although I had competed in several marathons since 2010, this was the first time I'd attempted an ultra. It did take a few days before I felt fully recovered and I gave it a full week before resuming gentle training again.

As a senior runner, I don't feel comfortable with the term Master runner. If you could see my race times, I'm sure that you would agree.

I am much more interested in how far I can run rather than how fast. However, as a senior runner, I am fascinated by just what sort of physical activity is possible as the body ages. Times change and our concept of *"Old Age"* is constantly being revised. I remember seeing books titled *"Staying fit at 50"* with pictures of a *"middle-aged"* couple in slacks and cardigan taking their dog for a walk. These days people into their 70s and 80s are running marathons, skydiving and taking part in all manner of vigorous activities which in years past would have been unthinkable.

I am very pleased to say that societies view of what counts as *"Old Age"* is changing and is due, in no small part, to people that are reading this book. People like **YOU!**

A contribution from: Glen Baddely, Ultrarunner 48 years old.

The notion of running anything more than a marathon in my early 20's was a non-starter, way beyond what I was capable of. As you get older you can rationalize the issues better and realize its often your head that controls the outcome when the distances increase.

In our distant past, we were hunter-gatherers, and our bodies are designed to be physically active.

So, if an active 80-year-old has similar physiology to an inactive 50-year-old, it is the younger person who appears older than they should be, not the other way around.

What's interesting is that, while many people in their 80s and 90s may be starting to take it easy, 85-year-old track star Irene Obera is at the other end of the spectrum. Setting multiple world athletics records in her age category, she is one of a growing band of *"master athletes"* who represent the extreme end of what is physically possible later in life.

Nevertheless, the fact that our bodies age is undeniable. Our strength declines relatively, as we age. So, we need to pay more attention to what we eat and how much rest we get. But where are the boundaries? Is there a time when we become simply too old? 70, 80, 90, 100? Fauja Singh BEM is a British Sikh centenarian marathon runner of Punjabi Indian descent.

His current personal best time for the London Marathon is 6 hours 2 minutes. This gives someone like me, i.e *more interested in how far I can run rather than how fast,* an awful lot of encouragement.

Of course, this question is relative. Someone who has been taking part in continuous vigorous physical activity since they were young has a far better chance of continuing into old age than someone taking up vigorous activity for the first time in later life. Particularly so if, up until that point, they had been living a sedentary lifestyle.

Next time you're out training and that voice inside your head tell you that you've set yourself an impossible goal - think of John Starbrook. At 87, he was the oldest finisher at the 2018 Virgin Money London Marathon.

The oldest person ever to complete the London Marathon was **Fauja Singh** who completed the course in 2004 aged 93.

But of course, it's not just runners that have set age records.

Martina Navratilova became the oldest main draw Wimbledon tennis champion at the age of 46 and Soccer player, Kazuyoshi Miura, 52, of Yokohama FC is the world's oldest professional footballer.

Still think you might be "Too old to ultra?"

How about Otto Thaning? Thaning became the oldest person to swim the English Channel at 73. He said that he had wanted to show what older people are capable of if they look after themselves.

He took the title from Australian Cyril Baldock, who only last month swam the channel three months shy of his 71st birthday.

Or, 71-year-old Linda Ashmore was the oldest woman to do the same thing and in 2017. Robert Marchand cycled 14 miles in an hour at the age of 105, setting a record in the process.

And that's without considering the incredible ultramarathon runners mentioned elsewhere in this book. Our peers and society in general often play a big part in how we view ourselves concerning where we fit in the World. We, humans, are very judgemental. There is a famous Zen saying that says:

"The World is not the way we think it should be"

Running over a certain age provokes that reaction in some people. I've lost track of the number of people that tell me why they don't run or that I need to find other sports because running *"at my age"* is bad for my health. I dare not tell them that I had a heart attack some years back. They would go into meltdown.

There are many well-documented stories about older runners. Gene Dykes is 70 and retired, but rather than spending his days pottering in the garden he's opted to run multiple ultramarathons and sub-3hour marathons. In 2019 he completed the 218-mile Delirious W.E.S.T. ultramarathon in Australia in 101 hours.

Dykes, from Philadelphia in the USA, has run 144 marathons and ultra-marathons since taking up running aged 56. His race schedule for 2019 would make many pro athletes' shudder: it includes five marathons (including Boston and New York) and 13 ultras.

He lives by his mantra 'Just run'. *"I say to everyone, 'Just run – don't search for magic bullets, just get out there and run.' They say, 'Can I do a 50-miler?' Just run! Why agonize over it? If you don't finish, so what?"*

Dykes's extraordinary running journey began when, aged 56, a friend asked him if he likes to go for a run. He'd run occasionally in the past but never raced. But after training for, and completing, a seven-mile race, the fire was ignited. He entered more events and slowly built up to New York Marathon, where he ran a not-too-shabby 3.43, aged 58.

"Once I started doing the races, I tried to beat my previous times – I've always been competitive," he says.

Incredibly, his times began improving with age. He improved his PB to 3.14 but then became frustrated after his next marathon dropped to 3.29.

Dykes's advice to anyone thinking about taking up running is to find what works for you.

"Some people like solitude, some people like to run with a gang, some like roads, some trails, some track..." he says. *"The important thing when you take up running is to remember there's nothing worse than being out of shape".*

"And don't worry about anyone else, just beat what you did last week. That's an easy measure of progress."

Great advice, I think. Slowly making forward progress, one step at a time.

As we get older, we maybe need to learn to pick our battles. Perhaps as an older athlete, you are never going to make massive improvements for your half marathon again, it's possible that genetics and the aging process simply won't allow it. However, as an older runner, somewhere between 13 and 25 miles, your strength (both mental/physical) comes into play. It's a tortoise and hare situation.

Still think you might be "Too old to ultra?"

Here is a little bit of research for you. Contributor, ultra-runner **Ian Thomas** has a few people he would like you to check out.

Ian Thomas Male age 60

Ian has run many ultras including the big UK canal races like The Grand Union Canal Race (GUCR) 145 miles, Liverpool to Leeds 130 miles, the Centurion Grand Slam of 100 milers and Spartathlon 153.4 miles for the last 4 years.

I strongly suggest that for anyone still in any doubt that older athletes can't compete should check out athletes such as Ivan Bretan - Sweden, Jan Spitael (aka Yannis Thirio)-- Belgium, Zigniew Malinowski - Poland, Martin Ilot Uk, Russ Bestley Uk, Andy Ives Uk, Pete Johnston Uk, Ann Bath UK, James Ellis UK, Mimi Anderson Uk, Emmanuel Psaradakis (Greece) All of the above are 50 plus and some have set National and International records.

Chapter 5.   Ultra-heroes

I do believe that, given the right preparation and training, anyone can complete an ultra-marathon. Particularly so, if your ambitions are confined to one of the shorter events, 32 to 50 miles. I've explained how it's all about getting the miles under your belt and not how fast you cover them. Many strategies can be employed to get you around, some people run a mile then walk a mile. Some give themselves a certain amount of time running, broken up with short periods of walking. I'll talk about a bit more about these techniques in future chapters. However, some people really do *"run"* an ultra, usually only walking very briefly or when traveling through checkpoints to hydrate and top up with food.

These men and women are what I'd call Ultra heroes. Here are a few of my favorites.

Kilian Jornet

Kílian Jornet Burgada was born on the 27th October 1987 in Sabadell, Catalonia. 1987, God that makes me feel old. Killian started as a skier but progressed to ski mountaineer and long-distance runner. He has been described as a marketing man's dream – good looking and talented, yet humble. He is a six-time champion of the long-distance running Skyrunner World Series and has won some of the most prestigious ultramarathons, including the Ultra-Trail du Mont-Blanc, Grand Raid, the Western States Endurance Run and the Hardrock Hundred Mile Endurance Run.

Ultra-competitive over everything from 1km to 200 miles Kilian has done it all.

The ability to be at the top of two sports and pursue unique projects has given rise to a completely new way of looking at running. He has utilized the rise of social media in a very clever way by bringing us stunning images without an overtly commercial message. Like a good wine, he seems to be getting better with age. At the time of writing, Jornet holds the fastest known time for the ascent and descent of Matterhorn, Mont Blanc, Denali, and Everest.

Recommended reading: Run or Die: The Inspirational Memoir of the World's Greatest Ultra-Runner by Kilian Jornet

Scott Jurek

Scott Gordon Jurek was born on October 26, 1973. Scott Jurek was probably the first ultramarathoner that I heard about and I read his book, Eat and Run from cover to cover. Scott hails from the U.S.A and throughout his career, has been one of the most dominant ultramarathon runners in the world. Scott has won many of the sport's most prestigious races multiple times, including the Hardrock Hundred (2007), the Badwater Ultramarathon (2005, 2006), the Spartathlon (2006, 2007, 2008), and the Western States 100 Mile Endurance Run (1999–2005). In 2010, at the 24-Hour World Championships in Brive-la-Gaillarde, France.

Jurek won a silver medal behind the Japanese ultramarathon runner, Shingo Inoue and set a new US record for distance run in 24 hours with 165.7 miles (an average pace of 8 minutes and 42 seconds per mile). Named one of the greatest runners of all time, Scott Jurek is simply a living legend.

Recommended reading: North. Finding My Way While Running the Appalachian Trail: Finding My Way While Running the Appalachian Trail12 Apr 2018 by Scott Jurek and Jenny Jurek

Dean Karnazes

Dean Karnazes born Constantine Karnazes on August 23, 1962 and is an American ultramarathon runner. His book, Ultramarathon Man: Confessions of an All-Night Runner was another of the books that I devoured when I first got interested in ultrarunning. TIME magazine named him as one of the *"Top 100 Most Influential People in the World."* Men's Fitness hailed him as one of the fittest men on the planet. He certainly is that. Dean has run across Death Valley in 120-degree temperatures, and he's run a marathon to the South Pole in negative 40 degrees. Dean also Ran 3,000-miles Across America from the coast of California to New York City and Ran 50 Marathons, in 50 US States, in 50 Consecutive Days.

Dean has won Badwater and the 4 Deserts Race Challenge. It's been said that Dean has pushed himself harder than most on a journey of self-discovery with very little reference points guiding him. Dean brought a niche pursuit to the masses and turned has it into a sport for the masses.

Recommended reading: Ultramarathon Man: Confessions of an All-Night Runner, The Road to Sparta: Running in the Footsteps of the Original Ultramarathon Man and 50/50: Secrets I Learned Running 50 Marathons in 50 Days -- and How You Too Can Achieve Super Endurance! All by Dean Karnazes

Bruce Fordyce

Bruce Fordyce was born on the 3rd of December 1955 in Hong Kong and is a South African marathon and ultramarathon athlete. Bruce is one of the genuine *"old guard"* distance runners who was running ultras before there were ultras. He is best known for having won the South African Comrades Marathon a record nine times, of which eight wins were consecutive. He also won the London to Brighton Marathon three years in a row. He is the current world record holder over 50 miles and the former world record holder over 100 km. Bruce is a perfect example of a senior athlete still competing. In his 60s he is South Africa's greatest ultra-marathon runner.

His 50-mile record has sat unbroken for 21 years now. This sort of feat does happen in long distance running, but is less and less common every year, as the sport swells in popularity, intensity, and with new technology. Bruce Fordyce also stood against apartheid as a public figure, long before it was acceptable or safe to do so.

Yiannis Kouros

Yiannis Kouros was born on February 13th, 1956 in Tripoli, Greece and is another of the *"senior"* elite ultramarathon runners. Yiannis holds many men's outdoor road world records from 100 to 1,000 miles and many roads and tracks records from 12 hours to 6 days. At the time of writing his longest recorded run is 646 miles. Crazy right?

I have called a chapter of this book, *"It's all in the mind"* The correct mental approach to completing an ultra is vital. It is said that, of all ultra-runners, Kouros can access his mental strength to get through races. Yiannis it is a master of the mental game. His training consists entirely of track work.

He says that he never runs more than 10 to 12 Kilometres and breaks this down into even smaller runs. You might well wonder just when he does his long runs. He says that his races are his long runs, ha, ha. He admits that this training program wouldn't work for everyone.

He does have some great motivational sayings when it comes to his body and its response to pain. For example,

"The pain is the reality, but your mind can inspire you past it," and *"when other people get tired, they stop. I don't. I take over my body with my mind, I tell it that it's not tired and it listens."*

Emelie Forsberg

From the old to one of the new generations of ultrarunners, Emelie Tina Forsberg was born on 11th December 1986 and is a Swedish athlete specialized in Trail running (Skyrunning, Mountain running) and Ski mountaineering. Like Killian Jornet she has inspired many with her infectious passion.

Her love of life, which she daily shares via social media. Emelie has won repeated victories in different disciplines, including European and World Championships. The young Swedish runner has impressed since she came on the scene with her enthusiasm and energy and her incredible downhill speed over the roughest of terrain. Recently Emelie achieved yet another record. After establishing new speed marks in Monte Rosa and Mont Blanc in late June, she now possesses also the Fastest Known Time (FKT) in the Kungsleden Trail, in the Swedish Lapland. She completed the 450km trail in 4 days and 21 hours, beating the current FKT, held since 2017 by Norwegian ultrarunner Sondre Almdahl, who completed the trail in 6 days, 2h 51'*

Chapter 6.   I get knocked down,

Kings Forest Ultra – October 2015

After the disappointment of not completing Peddars Way, I decided to make my next attempt a little easier, although I'm not sure there is such a thing as an easy ultra. However, if such a thing does exist, then the Kings Forest has got to be a contender. Coming in at a little over 32 miles, approx. 50k, it falls firmly into the *"baby"* ultra-marathon category.

The Kings Forest is just 4 miles outside Bury St Edmunds, easily accessible from East Anglia, London, and the East Midlands. The route provides a wonderful traffic free course on forest tracks around the sight of an ancient Anglo-Saxon settlement.

The race is run in October, so usually, the weather is usually mild. The course runs through beautiful forest tracks and apart from a little incline at the end is flat.

These days, like a lot of running events, Kings Forest has been changed to accommodate distances other than an ultra. Since 2018, it's possible to enter a half or full marathon as well as the ultra. Runners can run one lap for the half marathon and two for the marathon. Ultrarunners will continue on to complete the 3rd lap. The course is marked and there are drinks stations approx. every 7 miles. The course is off road* and traffic free using footpaths and tracks across Breckland and in the forest.

When I competed in 2015, you could only do the ultra.

This was one of the few races I've done with my friend and contributor to this book, Charlotte (Charlie) Harwood. I wasn't in the best of shape to take on this race. I had completed a standard marathon in September and, since it takes anywhere up to a month for your body to recover, I was still feeling a little fatigued. However, the great thing about running with friends is that they do lift your spirit. I managed to stay with Charlie for a good way into the race before the dreaded cramp started to kick in. For me, cramp is an early sign that my muscles have not fully recovered. When this happens, you have no other remedy than to stop and stretch. Try to massage and knead away the cramp. Take some water and walk it off. If you are lucky and you go steady, you can gingerly start back running.

I was affected with cramp in various degrees for much of the latter part of the race. I'd stop and walk it off before being able to pick up the pace. I well remember, catching back up to Charlie's group and hear her say, *"Here he comes, keep going Steve"* Unfortunately after another mile or so, running at Charlie's pace, the cramp would *"bite me"* again and I'd have to reluctantly let her go.

However, after missing out on Peddars, there was no way that I wasn't going to finish Kings Forest. I persevered. I ran. I jogged, I walked, and I hobbled and finished the race duly completing the 32 miles.

I'm pretty sure that I was the last finisher. Frankly, I didn't care. In my experience, when you tell people that you have completed a race of 32, 40, 50 miles or more, very few people ever ask you where you came.

Chapter 7.   Where to start

As I mentioned previously, you would be well advised to have a few marathons under your belt before moving up to the ultra-marathon distances. However, if standard marathons are no longing challenging enough for you, and you're thinking about attempting an ultra, this chapter will help to get you started.

Contribution from: Glen Baddely, Ultrarunner 48 years old.

My advice to someone wanting to do an ultra is just start. Most people read 'ultra' and immediately conclude its impossible. Wrong! Yes, it's hard, yes it requires dedication, yes it will require you to train your body and mind, BUT it's not impossible.

If you can only run a mile, then a 5k is just as unachievable. Also, while there are cut-offs in many races, they are not geared towards the elite, so the achievement is in completing the event not the time it takes. I completed a 100miler is all that's required (if the cutoffs are made). I ran across a desert, completing this is the achievement.

Listen to your body*.... some require running daily in some form, others require rest days.... some have issues around joints that need managing, so less tarmac work. Ultras help: the vast majority are off road.... trails, grass, fields, towpaths.... more forgiving surfaces, so train on a similar mix. One to get used to it, and two to preserve your joints.*

Many people who attempt a marathon consider it to be the king of long-distance running. They view the 26.2-mile distance as the absolute limit of their ability. Once its over, people find themselves into two separate groups. They either set about planning next year's event to try and improve their time or they make a solemn pledge to never attempt such a distance ever again. If you are in the former camp, and since you are reading this book, I'm guessing that you are, then read on.

Contribution from: Nick Jones, Ultrarunner 48 years old. Start gradually, Rome wasn't built in a day, I have built up from 2-3 mile runs and it has taken a long time to be able to get to ultra/marathon running.

Go off too fast and you will get injured, a friend of mine is running a Marathon this year they didn't listen and now have an injury, 5 weeks before it starts.

Finding your race.

Listed below are just a few possible races that you might want to check out. I have selected ultras of around 50 miles give or take. I've also listed some web addresses where other similar runs can be found.

Peddars Way Ultra

You would expect this to be my first choice having taken on the challenge myself. At a total distance of 48 miles, this ultra runs from the Suffolk border to the North Norfolk coast with well-stocked checkpoints every 12.5 miles. Cut-off time is 12 hours and there is a partial cut-off time at Castle Acre checkpoint.

The minimum requirement for runners is to have a run at least one marathon in the last 12 months. First aiders will be present during the entire race.

A coach will be available to transport runners from the finish line (Holme Next the Sea) to the start of the race at Knettishall Heath.

Personal drinks can be sent to each checkpoint and a small drop bag can be transported to the Castle Acre checkpoint at 26 miles. Hot food and drink will be available at the finish line.

The mandatory kit will be checked during the race and no pacers are allowed.

Thames Trot

The Thames Trot is 50 miles along England's mightiest river. Highly recommended by Steve West because it is easy to run, has great organization and relaxed cutoffs. It is quite a long one to start with, but a reasonable fee and a good one to bring supporters to. A big, mixed field of runners for this one.

Round Ripon Ultra

Anne-Marie Lord was a fan of this one because of the great scenery. It is also a good one to test your navigation skills out on. It is a 35-mile route which includes a world heritage site, pretty Yorkshire villages, woodland tracks, and open moorland, and a Royal deer park. Entrance to the Round Ripon Ultra is very reasonable.

Kintyre Way Ultra Half

Recommended by Ultra doyenne, Angela N Brin. She says the Kintyre Way is good for beginners due to the generous cut-offs, which does away with one of the big worries for a newbie ultra-runner. Very pretty in good weather – and of course Scotland is famed for its weather! – and not too technical. It is 35.5 miles from Tayinloan to Campbelltown with 1300m of ascent. So, you get to give those climbing legs a stretch.

Centurion 50s

The Centurion South Downs Way 50 (SDW50) and North Downs Way 50 (NDW50) are good first ultras to consider. A 50-mile race may not sound beginner friendly, but Centurion races are brilliantly organized, with impeccable course-marking.

The race has well-stocked aid stations at regular intervals and friendly volunteers. The South Downs Way 50 (in April) and North Downs Way 50 (in May) both take in point-to-point routes on National Trails, with manageable amounts of elevation for those of us who aren't natural mountain goats.

Centurion does four 50-mile events (in addition to SDW50 and NDW50 there's Chiltern Wonderland 50 and Wendover Woods 50) so there's plenty for any budding ultra-runner to have a go at. Wendover Woods 50 is probably less suitable for a beginner (it has 3,050m of ascent) but the others are all ideal for a first 50 miler. There's a minimum entry requirement of having run a marathon in less than the cut-off time. Find out more about all the Centurion 50-mile races

The Lakeland 50

Fifty miles in the Lake District? A beginner's Ultra? This is not an easy run but it deserves its place because the cut off is 24 hours so it is achievable for anyone who can persevere. It is also through one of the most beautiful parts of England and the terrain and weather will probably both challenge you. You can do the Lakeland 50 solo, in a pair or a three. Long established, with excellent organization and a chance to mingle with the elite mountain

Chapter 8.   How to get it done

Preparation is key

As with many things in life, the preparation you make before an event often dictates the degree of success. Without a doubt the single biggest factor in completing an ultramarathon is preparation. I have completed many standard marathons over the years. At one time I was doing several a year. Sometimes, I went ahead and competed knowing that I was not in the best of shape. On one memorable occasion, I ran the Milton Keynes marathon two days after recovering from food poisoning. Not a good idea. The point is that my body and mind was quite accustomed to running 26 miles.

Leaving aside the fact that I would be slow, I knew that, even though I was not at 100% I could still *"get it done"*. You simply can't get away with that in an ultra – no matter how many you have done.

Unlike almost any other race, you cannot simply rock up to ultra and expect to complete it........

The distance will beat you.

Contribution from: Nick Jones, Ultrarunner 48 years old.

Look at training plans, there are loads out there and they are worth their weight in gold, don't just pick one, have a look at a few mix and match but take advice.

Hit the gym.

Your typical marathon runner will often be carrying very little body fat. The typical image is of a tall lanky, thin as a rake athlete looking like they badly need a decent meal. Many years ago, distance runners simply *"Ran"* to train. Today most runners include gym work in their training. I would suggest that for anybody considering taking on an ultra, hitting the gym is a must.

Pick your battles.

Start early and give yourself plenty of time to train and prepare. Choose a race that suits you in terms of distance and location. Most regular ultramarathons will have their next year's races already planned and in the calendar.

I'd recommend giving yourself somewhere between 10 to 12 months to get ready. Don't allow yourself to be ambitious the first time out. There is nothing wrong with your first outing being a modest 30 odd mile event.

Contribution from: Glen Baddely, Ultrarunner 48 years old.

Now I've got older, I've learned to pick my battles. I'm never going to dip below 1:35 for a half marathon again, genetics and aging process won't allow......BUT my best for a marathon is 4:05. Somewhere between 13 and 25 miles, my strength (both mental/physical) come into play. It's the tortoise and hare situation, I believe it's a target I can aim for.

Also, the notion of running anything more than a marathon in my early 20's was a non-starter, way beyond what I was capable of. As you get older you can rationalize the issues better and realize its often your head that controls the outcome when the distances increase.

It also helps to realize where you 'fit' in this whole running thing. Before I started doing Ultra's I thought around 10 % of the population in the UK will have run a marathon before.

The reality is 1%. Looking at 50miles its 0.1%, and for 100miles....0.001%. Now that puts it into perspective.

Injuries are a key part in getting older.....I've not found I've struggled any more or less than I used to, BUT whenever I'm injured I may as well write off at least 2 weeks of training, things that sorted themselves overnight now take days/weeks to shrug off, and mentally it can be hard.

I tend to run with people around my age (+/- 5 years) just because we talk and run, and we share problems / have a laugh as we go. Some are friends from schooldays, others just happen to live in the same street. Some are happy to run a marathon, others keen to do Ultras with me.

I've learned that the key is not to run as much as I used to. Typically, I have 2 rest days now and use a cross-trainer at the gym for 2 days combined with weights.

So, I run 3 days a week, a shorter tempo session during the week, then Saturday and Sunday, which always includes a long session (up to 30miles depending on what I'm training for), and a follow-on session on the Sunday of about 50% of the long distance. This gives less 'hammer' on the knees over the week. I run between 100-140 miles month +gym sessions + races, not incl. parkruns (I normally race 4 times a year, a shorter time specific race, 2 Ultras up to 50 miles and an A race which is the focus, either longer or a stage race).

I amended this way of training when I suffered medial ligament issues after a run (still don't know how), but it sidelined me for 12 weeks.

Time on your feet.

There is an old saying in marathon training, *"it's all about time on your feet"* At the end of this book you will find a transcript of a Podcast that I gave a while back. In it, I describe a training routine that I do when preparing to run an ultra. **I WALK!** Yes, that's it. I walk. I pick a route of between 20 miles and 25 miles. I try to make it one large loop. That way you don't face the agony of passing your house several times on your way around for three or four more laps. I set out in the morning knowing that I'll be out all day, (time on your feet). I walk, sometimes I jog but mostly I walk. Frankly, there are only two reasons that I might run. One to relieve boredom.

The other is if I have miscalculated the time needed to complete the loop. If it's getting late, then I will pick it up and run, simply to get back home.

I find this a great mental and well as physical exercise to do. It can be very lonely running an ultra and to be comfortable with your thoughts is a very useful skill to develop. It's probably the only training that I do when walking is harder than running.

Explore your route.

If you can recce an area before you run your ultra, then do take the opportunity. It's not always possible, particularly when you have far to travel. At the very least inspect the route as best you can use maps of the area.

An ultra is not like a 10k or even a marathon. I have driven myself to a marathon location, never having competed in that race before. I've run the race and then driven myself back home again. The route is well marked and there will be marshals at regular intervals around the course. Not so with an ultra. Having invested a lot of training time getting yourself in good physical and mental strength, isn't it worth investing a bit of time in exploring the route? In the Podcast transcript at the end of this book, I explain how I recce a typical ultra.

Final preparation.

When you run an ultramarathon, two main aspects can have a great bearing on the performance - the training you have done leading into the race, and secondly the mental aspect of the race.

If you have done all the training you have set out to do in the months before the race, and you are on the start line with no injuries, then you are halfway there to having a great race. You shouldn't be thinking negatively. There is nothing more you could have done up until this point.

Chapter 9.   Nutrition

Ahh, nutrition. To carb or not to carb. Carbohydrate is the most efficient source of energy for athletes, right? It doesn't matter what sport you play; carbs are king. They provide the energy that fuels muscle contractions. Once consumed, carbs break down into smaller sugars (glucose, fructose, and galactose) that get absorbed and used as energy. Any glucose not needed right away gets stored in the muscles and the liver in the form of glycogen. Once these glycogen stores are filled up, any extra gets stored as fat.

Glycogen is the source of energy most often used for exercise. It is needed for any short, intense bouts of exercise from sprinting to weightlifting because it is immediately accessible.

Glycogen also supplies energy during the first few minutes of any sport. During long, slow duration exercise, fat can help fuel activity, but glycogen is still needed to help break down the fat into something the muscles can use.

Stay off the Sugar Train as long as you can.

Most of us run on sugar. We consume tons of it throughout the day. And since we now live a go-go-go society, we're in a constant state of stress that tells the body it needs to burn sugar to help keep us going. You have about 160,000 calories' worth of energy in your body at any given time. Only 4500 to 5500 calories are in the form of sugar. A lot of that is reserved for your brain and nervous system.

That doesn't leave much for distance running. The way most of us run, those sugar reserves are quickly depleted, at which point the options are (a) stop running; or (b) refuel with more sugar. If you don't do one of the two, your body physically shuts down, as a way of hanging onto what little sugar it has left for brain function. And that's what is often referred to as *"Hitting the Wall"* or what runners often call a *"bonk"*.

However, when it comes to long distance running, as an athlete, you may want to consider training your body to burn fat instead of carbohydrates. While carbohydrates provide an efficient fuel source, stores are limited. However, stores of fat provide twice the energy at nine calories per gram of fat.

There are a few main ways to encourage your body to burn fat preferentially when running and there has been some interesting research which is freely available online.

But can Keto work for you, as an older athlete, running an ultra?

Well, I'm fascinated by the potential benefits as an older endurance athlete. I've experimented with Keto (very low-carb, high-fat) diets, and I've learned, that once my body is in a fat-adapted state, I'm *"virtually bonk proof."* It is sometimes hard for me to get keto adapted. However, once there, I have found that I can exercise for hours on end just using just body fat for fuel. Most of us can store at least 40,000 calories as fat. I have found that I can make use of that supply quickly and easily.

On the other hand, our bodies can only store about 2,000 calories of carbohydrates. Therefore, so many endurance athletes *"hit the wall"* and constantly need to replenish glucose stores with gels and sugary drinks.

There are several studies which highlight the benefits of following a keto diet for older people generally.

Insulin resistance: Some senior people are prone to weight issues and are dealing with insulin-related conditions like diabetes. Serious, since diabetes can lead to things like vision loss, kidney disease, and more.

Bone health: Osteoporosis, in which reduced bone density causes bones to become fragile and brittle, is one of the most common conditions seen in older men and women.

Inflammation: For many people, aging includes more pain from injuries that happened at a younger age or joint issues like arthritis.

Being in ketosis can help reduce the production of substances called cytokines that promote inflammation, which can help with these types of conditions.

Nutrient deficiencies: Older adults tend to have higher deficiencies in important nutrients such as **Iron:** deficiency can lead to brain fog and fatigue. **Vitamin B12:** deficiency can lead to neurological conditions like dementia. **Fats:** deficiency can lead to problems with cognition, skin, vision, and vitamin deficiencies.

Vitamin D: deficiency cause cognitive impairment in older adults, increase the risk of heart disease and even contribute to cancer risk

The value of a Keto diet for Aging

Keto foods deliver a high amount of nutrition per calorie. This is important because the basal metabolic rate (the number of calories needed daily to survive) is less for seniors. However, they still need the same amount of nutrients as younger people.

A person age 65+ will have a much harder time living on junk foods than a teen or 20-something whose body is still resilient. This makes it even more crucial for seniors to eat foods that are health-supporting and disease-fighting.

Ok, so it seems that there are definite health benefits associated with following a keto diet. But how does that relate to the older endurance athlete as opposed to your *"average"* older person? It's a fact that, as we age, our muscles become less responsive, i.e. the anabolic effects of protein and exercise. It gets harder for us to build muscle as we get older. Eating more protein can help reduce muscle loss or at least off-set this anabolic resistance. People who take on more protein can maintain around 40% more muscle compared with those who eat very little protein. So, it may be that taking carbs out of the equation and increasing protein and healthy fats can be a positive factor.

The type of fat you consume may also make a difference in your ability to build muscle. There is convincing evidence that, in terms of preserving muscle mass, omega-3s become more important as we get older.

Low blood levels of vitamin D are common across all age groups and it can become much more of an issue as we age. Our skin's ability to produce vitamin D from UV light diminishes. Studies have shown that low levels of natural UV may reduce muscle function and strength as well as adversely affecting performance. So, making sure that we get enough levels of vitamin D whether from sun exposure, diet or supplements becomes more important for optimal performance as we age. The best dietary sources include oily fish, egg yolk and liver.

The Government recommends a 10 microgram (400 IU) supplement of vitamin D3 during the autumn and winter months (between October and April in the UK).

The debate around keto and endurance sports is heated. The transition to keto is not necessarily an easy one. If you're a very active person, the drop-in performance you'll see might be discouraging.

As I've mentioned, I've had several attempts at becoming keto adapted. Each time I've found it hard. While the length of time it takes to **adapt** to a **keto diet** varies, I've found that the process usually begins after the first few days. However, it can take quite a while longer to feel the benefits.

During the transition, I found training hard and I was constantly fatigued. However, once adapted I got positive results.

There is lots of good reading out there outlining the pros and cons of keto-adaption

Chapter 10.   It's all in the Mind

Train for Toughness

Your power and fitness are important, but you also must develop your toughness by proactively exposing yourself to discomfort or uncertainty. This means training in the rain or when it's ridiculously hot or blowing like a tempest. It means getting comfortable eating whatever's available rather than stressing over a perfect nutrition plan. The more you can embrace discomfort and uncertainty in training the better prepared you will be to work through it in competition.

So, what does it take for you to reach your potential as an athlete? Is it between you and the course, you and the clock, or between you and your mind?

Success in endurance sports is all about mental strength. The ability to handle the pain and fatigue of oxygen debt. It's about your ability to master the limits that you think you have.

Are you mentally tough as an athlete? Is mental training an active part of your training? Do you know how to consistently harness the power of your mind to lift the level of your performance?

Are you the kind of athlete who beats themselves long before the race's finish?

One of the big pluses as an older person is that age has taught us to be resilient.

One of the first mental demands that must be tackled has to do with motivation. As you age, do you still have the desire to do what's necessary to achieve success? You may have the goal, but do you still have the drive? That energy to keep you focused and moving forward through necessary daily training?

We have the why, do we still have the will?

Contribution from: Nick Jones,
Ultrarunner 48 years old.

Yes, it's all in the mind, we ran 30 miles in training for 56.7. The rest wasn't physical it was our minds. It was telling us we can't do the distance. At the end I could have carried on as my mind just stopped telling me I couldn't make it once I crossed the line, get over the mental side of distance running and the physical comes easier.

As we age, we often develop a better coping mechanism to handle competitive pressure. The ability of older people to reflect and put things in perspective helps to control nerves. Staying cool and calm is a mental skill that you can master with practice. Having life experience makes it easier.

My view is that, there are three important things for you to consider when thinking about taking on an ultra. In my opinion they are:

1) The ability to handle pain and fatigue

I believe that as older people, we have the strength and life experience to better control our focus when it starts to hurt. We have been here before. Perhaps not while running an ultra, but certainly at some point in our life. We handle the pain and don't crumble.

2) The ability to maintain concentration

Older people can focus and have a great ability to focus on what's important and block out everything else. Our mental skills in this area directly affect our ability to handle the pressure. **Been there, done that, got the T-Shirt.**

3) The ability to deal with setbacks.

Older adults are used to dealing with adversity, setbacks, and failure. We learn from our mistakes and move on. **What doesn't kill us makes us stronger.**

"When the going gets tough, the tough get going"

As the saying goes. Or, as one sports psychologist puts it, mental toughness is

"the ability to consistently perform toward the upper range of your talent and skill regardless of competitive circumstances."

Being mentally tough means that no matter what the challenge.

You're able to withstand the pain and suffering and perform to your best.

You are stronger than you think you are

As an older adult we are often a victim of our own doubts and mental uncertainties. When we are young, we just assume that we are invincible. We can do anything. As we age and the aches and pains creep up, we begin to have doubts. Let me tell you now. ***You are physically capable of much more than you think.*** And, what you are capable of is has as much to do with your mental strength as it does your physical capabilities. You can go beyond what your perceptions of tiredness or fatigue are. When your brain is telling you *"You're tired. And need to Stop."* It's your mental strength that's way more important than your physical limitations.

Some training suggestions for mental toughness

I talk in another section of this book about some training that I do which helps me enormously mentally. It involves being out all day. While I'm out, I practice visualization. I imagine that I'm competing in an ultra and *"must"* finish. I practice little mind tricks. I really like, *"Run the mile that you are in"* in other words, focusing on the *"now"* and breaking the run down into small chunks. If a mile is too long, then make it a half mile or a quarter. Or, from one streetlight to the next. Walking meditation is also something that I do. I alternate between, what I call constructive visualization, where I play out race day scenarios in my head, to pure mediation where I just try to empty my mind.

Either way, it really eats up the miles and you are mentally training yourself to push through the barriers you will certainly face in an ultra.

Contribution from: Charlotte (Charlie) Harwood. Multiple Marathon and Ultrarunner. GREAT BARROW ambassador

Charlie and her liferaft

I took up running in what most would say is late in life 30s. so I was never going to make the Olympic team. However, it wasn't until I started multi-day running that it became very apparent, I was a baby. I look around the room and the average age is easily 55 and they have more than 3000 marathons collectively under their belt.

So, I start to become confused about my age category, and then over the events, it dawned on me. I am an older competitive runner and a young endurance eventer.

Most marathon/ultrarunners get to a stage where they stop competing (they feel that they are no longer competitively capable) and become an event runner. The difference is the achievement is the <u>completion</u> of the event and not the <u>competition</u> of the event.

For me, It's all about the training. When I have the time to train and the will power to push myself, I can produce 4 hours 30mins consecutive days and know that I still have a little in the tank. When I'm busy at work and run down by life I'm slower.

So, am I being thrashed by younger and older runners because young people want to train, and older people have the time to train and feel like they need to fight off ever increasing age and the health problems that come with lack of exercise?

So, mental toughness. Is it all in the mind?

For me, the question is, is it the mental aspect that turns you into an event runner or your age and physical capability? Or is it a combination of both? This answer is so personal to the individual. For me, I have a medical condition that makes me fatigue and endures nerve pain and loses brain cognitive ability. This means, for me, it was always about completing the event rather than winning the event.

Others get to the stage where to enjoy the event they slow down and take in the area and the people. Others no matter the age will want to win and will push themselves on and often get a place. The more I think about it the more I know I can't be bothered to train harder than I need too, but when I do, I know that I achieve.

So, it's not so much age as personality. The body adapts to its training however the recovery I've noticed takes me longer and longer. To start with I put it down to my medical condition until I looked at my calendar. 21matathons a year would be draining but the following year 52 and the year after 64 adding in longer ultra-events.

It wasn't that my recovery was not as fast it was more like I didn't give myself recovery time and the balance was all wrong. My body was adapting and recovering faster than most people could hope for. My medical conditions felt under control and for the first time in ages, I could go a whole day without a nap!

I broke a small bone in my foot (stress fracture) on day four of the 10 in 10 (Great Barrow Challenge), carried on finished and spent 2 weeks with my foot up and then ran the race to the stones 100km. 10km from the end tiredness came on so much I felt like I was standing still.

I got to a checkpoint crawled onto a mat and slept for 45mins while doctors looked on desperately thinking of reasons to pull me out. 45mins later I woke up a different person had some soup and started running.

People who don't run will never understand why you want to run further and faster and more than you ran last time. It's something you must feel if you don't feel the need to run 100miles than no matter how fit and able you are you can't run 100 miles.

Nothing can prepare you mentally for your body begging you to stop at 45miles knowing you are not even halfway. The mental drive to keep the pace up when you have been running for 7 hours.

The tiredness creeps up on you like your shadow and it won't go, doubts about your ability to start eats at your confidence. Everything is starting it upset you. One shoe too tight, label in your shorts, the wind on your face, you're hot then you're cold. Some man walking his dog on the other side of the road feels like he is faster than you. All of this hits you and you start drowning in your negative thoughts. You are the only person who can keep yourself afloat during this time in your ultra.

Your only liferaft is your determination to finish.

It can be a real tug of war of emotions. Sometimes physically you won't cut off or you have an injury that rules you unable to go forward.

Sometimes I have had to cling to that life raft with only my nose out of the water refusing to let go.

So, what happens when you let go? You slowly sink, and it's incredibly slow. There is no joy in stopping, the pain does not go away the sun does not come out and dry up all the rain. You sit in a puddle of your thoughts, why did I stop?

Could I have gone on? have I let myself down, everyone must think that I am a quitter. Each thought makes the water rise again and there are only two options. Stop and let the water take you, you did your best but it's over.

Or try again and next time hold on to that life raft so much tighter than it would have to be a natural disaster to get you to let go.

Charlie is not an imposing athlete to look at. When you meet this lovely young woman your first impression is of a friendly, if somewhat, slightly eccentric, person. There is no sense of the courage, determination and "heart of a lion" that lay within. Charlie is simply a legend.

*The Great Barrow Challenge is the first and ONLY 10-day Multi Terrain event in the UK, it offers multiple events and routes (marathon 26.2 miles and Ultra's 32 miles) in the lovely Suffolk countryside just 8 miles from Bury St Edmunds and Newmarket. You choose any distance and route, but many people opt for the ultimate challenge, to run 10 marathons in 10 days. A feat which Charlie has accomplished more than once.

Chapter 11.   The BIG boys

I've spoken about how you might get started on your ultra-marathon adventure I have also suggested a few smaller events to get you started. However, at some point on your journey, you may be tempted to pit yourself against one of the big boys. The events listed here are truly entitled to all the accolades that are written about them. where ultra-marathons are concerned, these are most definitely the big boys.

The Marathon des Sables

The Marathon des Sables, or the MDS as it's sometimes referred to, is a six-day, 251 km (156 miles) ultramarathon.

In just six days competitors must cross parts of the Sahara Desert in Southern Morocco, running over or through endless dunes, rocky outcrops and across white-hot salt plains. The race distance equates to running approximately six regular marathons. Although many of the World's best ultrarunners compete in this most prestigious of races, every year hundreds of lesser mortals also face the challenge. Among these brave souls taking on this most demanding of ultras are to be found people who society might well label, too old to ultra.

The problem is somebody forgot to tell them that.

Think you're too old to take on The Marathon des Sables?

In 2015 Sir Ranulph Fiennes became the oldest Briton to complete the Marathon des Sables.

Sir Ranulph's record as the oldest male finisher didn't last long. Bill Mitchell, 73-year-old fitness fanatic from Derbyshire took the record a couple of years later, only for his record to fall to the redoubtable David Exell, 75. David claimed the record taking just six days to run more than 155-miles - approximately six marathons - across the vast expanse of sand in southern Morocco.

Where are the older female runners? You may well ask.

Despite hosting the race for over 28 years, Morocco still fails to attract female participants. Up until recent years, the MDS has tended to be a heavily male-dominated event and has particularly struggled to attract participation from women. In 2016, 15% of the field was female and there were only three Moroccan women out of a total of 973 finishers.

Admittedly, ultra-marathon participation, in general, tends to be weighted towards men but in other races, the divide is smaller and, in many cases, shrinking further all the time. The difference between male and female winning times is also notable. Whereas in many long distance and multi-day events you will find a gap of perhaps 10-20% between male and female times on average.

For MDS, the differential over the past five years has been more than 30%. There are numerous reasons for this, not least that the race requires runners to carry their kit – which is likely to be heavier in proportion to body weight for women. But the lack of *"serious"* female runners from Morocco – runners who might be more used to the terrain – is another. While there is yet to be an older female runner in the 70s age range, there are certainly "older" female athletes pushing the boundaries. Notable amongst these is 50-year-old French ultra-runner, Laurence Klein. Laurence is a triple winner of the Marathon des Sables; 2007, 2011 and 2012.

Still, think that you are Too old to ultra?

The Spartathlon

If the Marathon des Sables isn't to your taste, there is always the Spartathlon. Spartathlon is a 246-kilometer ultramarathon race held annually in Greece since 1983, between Athens and Sparta, the modern town on the site of ancient Sparta.

Spartathlon is the event that brings this deed to attention today by drawing a legend out of the depths of history. The idea for its creation belongs to John Foden, a British RAF Wing Commander. As a lover of Greece and student of ancient Greek history, Foden stopped his reading of Herodotus' narration regarding Pheidippides. Puzzled and wondering if a modern man could cover the distance from Athens to Sparta, i.e. 250 km, within 36 hours.

SPARTATHLON is a historic ultra-distance foot race that takes place in September of every year in Greece. It is one of the most difficult and satisfying ultra-distance races in the world because of its unique history and background.

I've been fortunate enough to have had the benefit of contributions from several great runners during the process of writing this book. All of them have provided valuable insight.

However, one runner stands out and his name is **Ian Thomas**. Ian has competed at the highest level and has taken on several of the so-called *"Big Boys"* including Spartathlon.

Comments on Spartathlon from Ian Thomas

Ian has run many ultras including the big canal races like GUCR 145 miked, Liverpool to Leeds 130 miles, the Centurion Grand Slam of 100 milers and Spartathlon 153.4 miles for the last 4 years.

"I managed to finish my 4th Spartathlon in 2018 carrying an injury with 50 miles still to go during a Medicane (A Mediterranean Hurricane) The worst weather Greece had ever seen in that race".

With Ian's permission, I have included an account of his 2018 race report. You can read the full story and follow Ian's story on his blog.

https://ultraian.wordpress.com which is well worth following.

Ian Thomas – Spartathlon 2018 Race Summary

"Following the second year of inconsistent training due to niggles I found myself lined up once again at the start of this amazing, iconic but brutal race.

This will be my fourth consecutive finish if I make it and there were some lofty expectations from fellow runners, but I knew I wasn't the same highly trained runner of 2016 (the last year I had a good run of decent performances)

So, I was cautious and hesitant about what expectations I should set myself.

I've said it many times before, but you must believe you will cross that finish line before you start or else you won't. It's not arrogance, it's just convincing yourself that you have it in you. It's easier to persuade your subconscious of this when you know you have put in the required training and you've had a run of successes, since success begets success.

Much more difficult when you've had neither for a while and this was my potential dilemma as I battled self-doubt about what I would deliver based on last 18 months or so.

Yes, I had a reasonable showing at Belfast 24hr and managed to somehow win the Essex 100 but, they were sub-par lacklustre performances.

I knew I couldn't expect to excel, and it would take all my experience and self-belief just to finish Spartathlon this year. I didn't set any expectations on time as I knew this would be foolhardy but obviously, this didn't mean I wouldn't try to do my best.

I decided therefore that I needed to be more cautious this year, so I planned to hold back in the hope of saving something for the last third. Not my usual strategy as everyone knows.

What I hadn't reckoned on though was being walloped by Cyclone Zorba which was to constrain my pace still further as I negotiated the torrential rain and ankle-deep floods on the roads.

Whether this compounded problems I was experiencing with an ankle injury I sustained around the 100 mile point I don't know but somewhere around the mountain, I started to experience real pain in my ankle which was so debilitating and obviously decimated my pace.

I'm notorious for going off fast and am constantly criticized for it but as I've stated before I believe that regulating my pace to be slower than what feels natural to me adversely affects my gait. Whether this is what happened this year or not I don't know as other variables were introduced this year, including different shoes, cooler temperatures, incessant rain and hidden ruts in the road concealed by flooding.

As it transpired it wasn't pretty this year as I had to basically trudge it in from around 35-40 miles out from Sparta. Not my idea of performance or indeed a run for that matter, as I did all I could just to finish this year, but hey I will confine it to history and move on.

All I wanted to do was finish and to take Gills hand to the King. I didn't care about anything else. I knew I couldn't do myself justice, but I hope to put that right if I can secure a place next year.

First, I need to make sure I earn the right to line up again at the Acropolis though and although I have a qualifier I need to try and renew my AQ, so it's back to Athens in January for the 24hr".

Ian Thomas is over 60. Do, if you don't think that you are too old to ultra and want to know more about Spartathlon, check out: https://britishspartathlonteam.org/

The Badwater 135 - "The World's Toughest Foot Race"

The Badwater Ultramarathon describes itself as "the world's toughest foot race". It is a 135-mile course starting at 279 feet below sea level in the Badwater Basin, in California's Death Valley, and ending at an elevation of 8360 feet at Whitney Portal, the trailhead to Mount Whitney.

It takes place annually in mid-July when the weather conditions are most extreme, and temperatures can reach 130 °F. Consequently, very few people—even among ultramarathoners—are capable of finishing this...

Think you're too old to take on The Badwater 135?

70-year-old Bob Becker reached the 14,505-foot summit of California's Mount Whitney, scrawled his name in the summit register, but didn't hang around to celebrate. He had been running for the previous 67 hours and 25 minutes—and he was still only halfway on his attempt at the Badwater Double.

The Double is a 292-mile out-and-back route through Death Valley, from Badwater Basin—North America's lowest point, at 282 feet below sea level—to the summit of Whitney and back.

Still, think that you are Too old to ultra?

The Western States 100

Approximately 100 miles (160 km), the Western States 100 course runs from Squaw Valley to Austin, California

It was once a horse race over 100 miles. One time a starter's horse refused to run, and the rider didn't want to put the animal through the ordeal – so he quite simply ran the 100 miles himself.

The following year there were three, maybe four crazy people who said, *'okay we'll run too'*.

It's a hugely prestigious race. Look out for the clips on YouTube with many times race winner Scott Jurek.

There is also a great movie worth checking out called Unbreakable. It follows four of the top ultra-marathon men on this amazing journey. Hal Koerner, two times defending Western States champion, Geoff Roes, undefeated at the 100-mile distance, Anton Krupicka, undefeated in every ultramarathon he has ever started and Kilian Jornet, the young mountain runner and two-time Ultra-trail du Mont-Blanc champion, from Spain.

The Western States takes place on trails in California's Sierra Nevada annually, on the last weekend of June. The race starts at the base of the Squaw Valley ski resort and finishes at the Placer High School track in Auburn, California.

Runners climb a cumulative total of 18000 feet (5500 m) and descend a total of 23000 feet (7000 m) on mountain trails before reaching the finish.

Because of the length of the race, the race begins at 5:00 A.M. and continues through the day and into the night. Runners finishing before the 30-hour overall time limit for the race receive a bronze belt buckle, while runners finishing in under 24 hours receive a silver belt buckle.

The race takes place annually in late June. Only serious ultra-runners need to apply.

Think you're too old to take on The Western States?

At 67 years of age, Ian Maddieson's consistent effort throughout the day to finish the 100-mile journey in 27:44:41. The New Mexico trail runner took home the *Oldest Male Finisher* award.

In 2015 along with 300-odd other runners, 70-year-old Gunheld Swanson set out from the Squaw Valley ski area, some 100 miles away by trail, at the start of the Western States 100 Mile Endurance Run.

She was hoping to cross the finish line, only a couple hundred yards away, under the 30-hour cut off, like the 252 runners before her. If she made it, she would be the oldest woman ever to finish the storied race.

But she was cutting it close – As she rounded the final turn, she had less than 100 meters to cover, with less than 20 seconds to do so

"I turned the corner and I saw the clock and I knew I had it," she says. *"All I had to do was maintain the momentum. And there it was."*

Swanson collected the Oldest female Finisher award.

That was Swanson's third finish at the Western States; her personal best is 25:40:28, set in 2005 at the age of 60.

Still, think that you are too old to ultra?

Chapter 12.   Are Ultras bad

A cautionary tale.

From my friend Ian Thomas again. An account of his bad experience attempting to qualify for Spartathlon 2019

"I risked running with an injury to auto qualify for Spartathlon 2019 which I achieved but it could well have killed me due to development of Rhabdomyolysis. This is caused by the kidneys being unable to remove the by-products of muscle breakdown quickly enough caused by intensive long exercise without enough hydration.

In my case, it wasn't so much that I neglected hydration any more than I had previously, but because I had run for 24hrs with an injury the volume of myoglobin released in to my bloodstream was huge, so even with the usual hydration requirements it wasn't enough to help my kidneys. I should have taken on more fluid in the last 4 hours but didn't realize of course that I had developed Rhabdomyolysis.

Thankfully all's well now. It was a reckless thing to do which I justified beforehand by the need to AQ for Spartathlon.....

I will never risk running with an injury again - not even for Spartathlon"

So, are ultra-marathons bad for your health? Well, I guess the honest answer is, yes, they can be. But, as Ian points out, he took a calculated risk by running with an injury. It's worth pointing out that Ian is a very experienced runner who knows his body well.

Running ultra-marathons can be bad for you, as can running marathons or running half marathons. So can any physical undertaking if done recklessly and without proper preparation.

In a past life, working as a sports development officer with a local authority, I spent an awful lot of time filling out risk assessment forms. Anyone familiar with these forms will know that there is a formula which balances risk versus likelihood.

For example, on a scale of 1 to 10, how likely is it that someone will trip over a piece of sports equipment etc, and if they do, what is the severity of the likely injury, on a scale of 1 to 10 with 10 being fatal.

In my humble opinion, life is not about avoiding risk. Life is about managing risk. Hopefully, up until this point, I have put in enough caveats and self-assessment suggestions to demonstrate my commitment to your safety. I am not suggesting that any older person, with little or no running experience, can just jump in and complete an ultra-marathon, or even a standard marathon.

My advice is to, PLAN. PREPARE. GET YOURSELF PHYSICALLY AND MENTALLY FIT. PLAN SOME MORE. PREPARE SOME MORE. BUILD A SUPPORT TEAM. PLAN AND PREPARE A BIT MORE FOR GOOD MEASURE. THEN GO FOR IT!

I firmly believe that age should not prevent us from challenging ourselves. I believe that with enough training and preparation, who knows what we can accomplish.

Where endurance running is concerned, there has been much consternation about health concerns.

In 2018 a national newspaper ran an article entitled *"When 26.2 miles just isn't enough – the phenomenal rise of the ultramarathon"*. It's a great article and well worth checking out. It quotes Lindley Chambers, chairman of the Trail Running Association, as saying, *"the ever-growing contrast between our normal, sedate lives and the feeling you get running an ultra.*

Being fully alive and on the edge is key to the sport's growing appeal. As the world becomes ever more sanitized and automated, where even cars drive themselves, a deep stirring grows to get out of our comfort zone, to feel something of our wilder selves".

"As our regular, mundane lives become ever more sedentary," he says, **"we have a need for something more."**

The article highlights a documentary called, The Barkley Marathons: The Race That Eats Its Young, one competitor in the 100-mile race puts it more bluntly:

"Most people would be better off with more pain in their lives."

Getting through the pain barrier, the wall, pushing beyond your limits, was once part of the appeal of standard marathons. But, according to ultrarunner Nick Mead, the feeling you get, the fabled runner's high, is proportionally bigger in an ultramarathon.

After completing his first ultra, Mead wrote:

"The race pounded me almost into submission before I broke through and was lifted on a wave of euphoria unlike anything, I've ever experienced ... an almost spiritual high."

Contribution from: Nick Jones, Ultrarunner 48 years old.

I had issues prior to running longer distances, if anything it has helped my situation, a lot of Sarcoids suffers give up and end up in a chair with oxygen, it can improve if you fight it and that's what I'm doing.

The older I seem to get, the lower my times seem to be getting, my 10K PB was in Feb 2019.

Yet, while it may bring a feeling of wellbeing, can running a hundred miles or more, often through the night and through challenging terrain, really be good for your body? In 2012, cardiologist-runners Carl Lavie and James O'Keefe caused a stir when they released a research paper that found that while moderate running was clearly healthy, those health benefits began to tail off and possibly even reverse if you ran *"excessively"*. Initially, they defined that as more than 2.5 hours a week – though after further research Lavie revised it to five hours a week. Ultrarunners, of course, undertake much more than that, often in a single day.

Lavie and O'Keefe's main concern was heart damage and hardening of the tissue around the heart brought on by extreme exercise. In a TED* talk on the subject, O'Keefe said that while exercise was one of the best medicines for good all-around health, *"like any drug, there's an ideal dose range. If you don't take enough, you don't get the benefits. If you take too much, it could be harmful. Maybe even fatal."*

Mark Hines is a professional adventurer, author, and an exercise physiologist. He shares some of the health concerns about ultrarunning.

* TED Conferences LLC is a media organization that posts talks online

"The biggest issue is permanent scarring of the heart tissue," he says. "Anyone middle-aged running a marathon or more is likely to develop some level of scarring, and it is irreversible."

For me, so much of what I do is focused on achieving balance. For sure, excessive mileage can have a detrimental effect and particularly excessive "Hard" running. However, Lavie and O'Keefe were accused of putting people off running and are now keen to stress that any exercise is better than no exercise.

Dr Andrew Murray, a sports and exercise medicine consultant at the University of Edinburgh, who once ran 4,300km over 78 days from John o'Groats to the Sahara Desert, emphasizes the point:

"There is a ceiling [in the amount of running you do] beyond which you start to lose the sweet spot health-wise. However, it is very difficult to do enough to return you to a greater risk than couch potatoes."

The problem with relating O'Keefe's study to ultrarunning is that he conflates the intensity and duration of exercise to define **"extreme"**.

Ultrarunning may, on the surface, seem to be extreme, but in practice, it is usually undertaken at a very low intensity – with walking forming a large chunk of most ultra-races for most competitors.

Indeed, Hines says he has started running longer races since he learned about the risk of heart scarring, because, he says, they are generally safer due to the lower intensity of effort.

In 2014, Dr. Martin Hoffman, professor of physical medicine and rehabilitation at the University of California, ran a more specific study on health issues related to more than 1,200 ultrarunners. He concluded that they were healthier than the non-ultrarunning population, with a low prevalence of virtually all serious medical issues, and that they had fewer sick days off work. *"At present,"* he told me, "there is no good evidence to prove there are negative long-term health consequences from ultramarathon running."

Contribution from: Glen Baddely,
Ultrarunner 48 years old.

Are ultramarathons bad for your health? In my opinion, if you approach them and train properly no, they are not. Attach a heart rate monitor and you will find that as you are moving more slowly you don't stress your heart with as many sharp rise/falls as tempo runs, and clearly fitness is good for a strong heart.

My motto, one life, live it.

But are ultramarathon runners doing it to be healthy? No one I spoke to cited that as the reason. Hoffman followed up his research with a fascinating question posed to another 1,394 ultrarunners: *"If you were to learn, with absolute certainty, that ultramarathon running is bad for your health, would you stop?"*

Seventy-four percent of runners responded: *"NO"*.

So, is running an ultramarathon detrimental to your health, particularly if you are an older athlete? On balance, providing that you have prepared well, I would say no. However, let's hear another cautionary tale from Glen Baddely.

Contribution from: Glen Baddely, Ultrarunner 48 years old.

One word of caution......with age doesn't necessarily come sense......I know I am driven to succeed, sometimes at the detriment of my body.

Two examples, while running across the Oman desert we were told checkpoints were about 6 miles apart to replenish water. I rationed my supply.... then ran out in the middle of dunes out of sight of where I thought the checkpoint was. I carried on for 30mins without water until I reached the CP, it was only after that I questioned how much further I would have carried on before I recognized it would be more prudent to withdraw...I'll never know because I finished it.

Another time my running buddy and I were around 93miles into a 100-mile race. We all know that due to dehydration our pee goes a darker shade of yellow and can contain traces of blood when dehydrated. I had been drinking plenty, and although my pee was a dirty yellow, nothing to be concerned about.... until I started to pee a deep red color. We looked at one another and I said....' I don't care I'm not stopping 7miles short, I'll deal with it later'. Again, we finished and the next time I went to the loo things were getting back to normal.

I found out later that when your body is pushed to the extreme, sometimes lactic acid can't escape and goes into your kidneys.... resulting in the blood. Common sense said, it's time to stop, I didn't.

Knowing what I know now it wasn't serious, but the point is I didn't know but still carried on. Maybe there is more James Cracknell in me than I give credit for!

I got close during the 100mile race to my limit physically, but if I had reached the finish line and they said.... another 5 miles please or its not official, could I have done it, slowly but yes, I could.

I haven't found my limit yet......until then I carry on.............

Chapter 13. Mental health

"I once lived a life almost ruled by anxiety, intrusive thoughts, and paralyzing fear. I spent years looking for the thing that would release me, and when I finally found it, it wasn't medication or therapy (although both helped). It was running. It gave me a feeling that there was a world out there beckoning me, promising hope; it gave me independence and the sense that I had reserves of strength that I wasn't aware of".

In researching this chapter of my book, I came across the quote above. It was amongst a selection of reference material I had collected for a separate book I'm writing called, *"Mental health in the long run"*.

I couldn't find the name of the person who said it or indeed where it came from at all. If you recognize the quote, then please let me know and I will give its author due credit. It is a powerful statement that perfectly embodies the link between running (physical exercise) and our mental health. It's generally acknowledged that physical activity is said to help mental health. At the very least– it boosts mood, relieves stress and improves sleep.

Running can also help use up some of the adrenaline caused by anxiety. People report positive relieve from panic attacks, intrusive thoughts and that looming sense of doom that comes from depression and anxiety.

The link between exercise and mental health is not new – in 1769, the Scottish physician William Buchan wrote that *"of all the causes which conspire to render the life of man short and miserable, none have greater influence than the want of proper exercise"*

One of the things that I've noticed, most of all, while writing this book is how the themes of resilience, recovery, and redemption seem to resonate with people.

I have had numerous letters and emails from runners and non-runners alike. All very happy to share their thoughts and opinions, particularly regarding how running impacts on their mental health and well-being. I've included a few reflections here.

The first is from my friend Charlotte Harwood, known by all as Charlie. Charlie is a legend and is quoted unashamedly in this book. I asked her what she looks for in a book about running and mental health.

From Charlotte Harwood

"What I enjoy about the books I read is knowing what rock bottom for them was, I want to know they cried as much as I do.

I want to know how they realized how they feel and when they noticed that their activities and mental health were related

I want to know what they thought of help or no help they had from professionals and fellow spots people.

I want to know that other people feel how I feel/felt".

Best wishes, Charlie

When researching for this chapter, I did a Google search using the search term – Running saved my life. It was incredible just how many stories came up. *"I **was** depressed and crippled with anxiety... Running saved my life."* Stories like:

I was depressed and self-medicating with alcohol, until running gave me the lifeline he desperately needed.

"Running Helped Me Overcome Anxiety and Depression."

And many, many more all with similar themes.

I have been very fortunate in that I have enjoyed reasonably good mental health in my life.

However, I can certainly relate to some of these stories. At the very least, and certainly, for me, the benefits I enjoy include building confidence, stress relief, and the attitude boost of the runner's high. Running is an aerobic cardiovascular exercise. It sends more nourishing blood to my brain, which can help you think more clearly. Running also releases my natural mood-elevating compounds. So, I usually feel good after my run.

There have been many interesting studies conducted over the years, designed to explore the relationship between running and particularly ultra-running and mental health.

Several of the studies looked at the ways ultra-running has impacted the runner's mental health and particularly around their engagement in ultra-running. They also looked at the promotion of healthy mental health practices, and the subject's dependency on ultra-running.

The studies looked to identify ways that ultra-running has impacted on the participant's mental health.

Ultra-running requires an individual to structure multiple aspects of their lives to be able to meet the demands that ultra-running has on the body and mind. Ultra-runners spend countless hours running, structure their diets and can spend a large amount of money for the sport.

Many of the studies found that the potential for ultra-running to have either a positive or negative impact on multiple aspects of an individual's mental health can make it a powerful activity to engage in.

A conclusion from some of these studies is that the potential that ultra-running must impact an individual's mental health. Ultra-running was found to have many aspects that may be beneficial to a participant's mental health including; the structure it requires, the social connections it fosters, the opportunity for self-exploration, and the physical benefits it gives. The participant appeared to find moments of catharsis and a release of emotional pain through their engagement in ultra-running.

So, while the jury is still out on the long-term effects of ultra-running on our physical health, there does seem to be evidence of positive wellbeing regarding our mental health.

Through all the studies a common theme has emerged in that.....

Participants in the studies talked about having a very positive association with running endurance events and finding them beneficial to their mental health and ability to cope with their depression.

Chapter 14.   Can athletes compete

In particular, can "older" athletes compete? Well, I'm afraid that it's an undeniable fact that, no matter how fit you were as a younger athlete, eventually age catches up to us all. As a 60 plus athlete, I can feel my body slowing down. When I first get out of bed, my legs ache as I walk stiffly downstairs. Sitting down and getting out of a chair, I'm inclined to occasionally make what my wife calls *"old people noises."* When I finally get out of the door to begin my run, I have heavy legs which take increasingly longer to shake out as each year passes. I need to take a much longer warm up before starting my run proper. I find that, because my recovery takes longer, I can no longer run every day.

I don't respond well to as many hard training days or as many hours of intense training as I once did.

Despite my sorry tales of aches and pains, is it possible for me and older athletes like me to keep running well both in training and races?

YOU BET IT IS.

It seems, getting older doesn't necessarily mean getting slower. Many world-class endurance athletes perform at their best in their late 30s and early 40s. But how about athletes in their 50s and 60's? Getting older means becoming smarter and more efficient with your training. The older you get, the smarter you need to be.

That means learning to respect your body as it ages, which often means changes in your warm-up, training, and recovery. Get these right and you can continue to run and compete well into the later stages of your life.

Here are a few necessary changes I have had to make as I've gotten older.

I need a longer warm-up—both in training and races.

In truth, I've generally needed a reasonable amount of time to warm up even as a younger athlete. However, it now definitely takes me longer to get my engine up to speed. I must allow a long and easier warm up. A run may start with a 2-mile walk run with some stretching added. The periods of walking are less about catching my breath and more about raising my heart rate slowly.

Allowing my body time to get going is key.

In the beginning, I felt a bit stupid going so slowly and constantly having to walk. However, I read an article about how the Kenya runners train. The article said that African runners begin their training sessions very slowly, often at an easy jog and gradually increase their pace. They say it's like slowly bringing water to the boil. When it comes to a race, I give myself up to 30 minutes of easy warm-up running before I feel race ready. Then, once I'm warmed up, I'm ready to go!

Think about your training to reduce volume.

I like serious training. But, as I've gotten older, I've tried decreasing the volume.

I love my hard runs, but my body simply gets too fatigued to respond if I do too many without rest. Recently though, I've been experimenting with increasing the volume but reducing the intensity. So, more runs but at a much-reduced pace.

Structure more recovery days between days of intensity.

I don't respond well to too many days of intensity each week anyway. My body can't recover and respond in time for the next hard run. So, I either allow a complete day of rest between hard runs. Taking lighter workouts between each heavy run allows me to absorb the load, adapt and recover, ready to go again.

Nutrition, sleep, and overall well-being are essential!

As a young man, I could eat whatever I wanted, get by on very little sleep and still get up every day to perform. As I've gotten older, that simply is no longer the case. The older you get, the more you need to treat your body with care. Nutrition, hydration, and sleep become essential to recovering well and performing at your best. There is lots of good research out there regarding nutrition and sleep particularly. It is the latest piece of the jigsaw regarding better performance for elite athletes and is vital if you wish to keep performing well as you age.

The role these things play can't be understated. Be mindful about your eating and sleeping and it will pay dividends. As with many things in life, it's all a question of balance.

There is an old song from the 1950s. I think it's called *"Son of a Gun"* It has a line which goes, *"Lucky, lucky, lucky me. I'm a lucky son of a gun. I work 8 hours, I sleep 8 hours, which leaves 8 hours for fun."*

Ah, if only life was that simple.

Contribution from: Nick Jones

I tried anything while training to get the right balance, the best thing I found that works for me, is gels and protein shakes, I have a high protein shake after every run to recovery and during my runs take gels (SiS), keep my food/diet normal to what I regularly eat so not to upset my stomach.

Contribution from: Glen Baddely

I've learned that its key not to run as much (as in as many days a week as I used to). Typically, I have 2 rest days now and use a cross-trainer at the gym for 2 days combined with weights.

So, I run 3 days a week, a shorter tempo session during the week, then Saturday and Sunday, which always includes a long session (up to 30miles depending on what I'm training for), and a follow on session on the Sunday of about 50% of the long distance. This gives less 'hammer' on the knees over the week. I run between 100-140miles a month +gym sessions + races not incl. park-runs (I normally race 4 times a year, a shorter time specific race, 2 Ultras up to 50 miles and an A race which is the main focus, either longer or a stage race).

I amended this way of training when I suffered medial ligament issues after a run (still don't know how), but it sidelined me for 12 weeks

Monitor your body and check out new technology

As I've become older, I pay much more attentive to my overall *"well-being"* I pay close attention not only to what my body feels like and regularly test my blood pressure and oxygen saturation using a finger monitor

For the serious older athletes, you can check out a device called the Ember Sport. This device measures 10 key metrics in less than a minute using an LED light finger sensor. You use it twice a day to capture hemoglobin, pulse rate variability, pulse rate, respiratory rate, pleth variability index, perfusion index, oxygen saturation, carbon monoxide, oxygen content, and methemoglobin.

It helps athletes track their sleep wellness and overall emotional wellbeing. It's a key indicator to identify If you are overtraining, dehydrated or potentially getting sick.

Nick Jones,

My times are coming down, I know this will stop at some point but that won't stop me trying or running, the benefits are too great and anyway we oldies have our own age brackets in running, while not run the fastest marathon aged 100. Running isn't always competing against the other runner; it's about competing against yourself and if you like the improvement or even where you are in your running that should be enough. I love running and my family love me to run.

Chapter 15. Where to next

I often compare my running to a game of snakes and ladders. I plan out my running goals for the year and set my training schedule accordingly. As I progress with my training, I slowly climb up the *"ladders"*. Regrettably, at some point, I will hit a setback. My training will stall, due to work commitments, injury or sickness or a combination of all three and I will slide inexorably down a *"snake"*. The problem is that the older I get, the *"ladders"* seem to be getting shorter and the *"snakes"* longer. The upshot of this is that progress towards optimal fitness takes longer as does my recovery.

A major goal is to complete The Stour Valley Path Ultramarathon. The SVP100 is a 100km (62 miles) long footpath in England. It starts in Newmarket (Suffolk) and ends in Cattawade, a village near Manningtree (Essex). The SVP100 covers almost the entire length of a well-marked trail and is one of the longest point to point races in East Anglia. The path is particularly notable for the beauty of the scenery. The event takes place in August and my target is the 2020 race. This gives me approx. 18 months to prepare. I've decided on this amount of time to fully prepare. If all goes according to plan, I'll complete the 62 miles at the age of 68 and I'll be pretty darn happy with that. Part of my preparation will include competing in several halves and full marathons, probably Mablethorpe in October 2019, Milton Keynes in May 2020 and at least one or more other early in 2020.

The SVP100's starting point is quite close to where I live so it makes the logistics of getting there a whole lot easier. It also means that I can dedicate a few weekends before the race, researching and running part of the route.

One of the other events I've promised myself next year is to compete in the Great Depression, otherwise known as the Great Barrow Challenge

This event has been mentioned several times in this book and great insight is provided here by my friend and contributor Charlie Harwood.

The great depression!

Most people know me as the GREAT BARROW ambassador, I'm always there and I'm happy to be there. The friendly family atmosphere all sitting on the sofas chatting. It's a mix of people that have run 700 marathons and those running the first. One of the big events each year is the 10 marathons in 10 days the only multi-train single loop of its kind and as it should be its brutal and challenging. I have cried, performed PBs, taken people round on their first marathon. Been dragged around. Hurt so much I thought I'd never walk again. Endured heat that is too much to run in and rain that has washed out footpaths as well as our campsite.

It's my favorite 10 days of the year. You meet new people and experience highs and lows, disappointment, determination. Comradery.

These people you will see at other races and greet like lost family or when running give the nod that says that's one of the family. All in a confined campsite with a small group of 50 people, who in a very small space of time you will sit almost on top of before a shower, share food with someone whose name your too tired to remember.

Hug people that yesterday made you cry. Get lost, laugh about other people getting lost. So why is it the great depression?

Last year's veteran 10 in 10 lots where arriving and I looked over and shouted "so are you ready for the great depression?" everyone laughed apart from a newcomer who asked if the 10 days was that bad to which everyone replied no it's the most wonderful 10 days of the year. He looked confused as he sat down. I explained to him you do the 10 days and it's amazing such an achievement. You go home you rest for a day and recover. You get up on Monday morning and you miss your new friends, eating breakfast together. Joking around. You look at your watch and said I would be at race briefing now or at checkpoint one. Then reality hits you, it's over you did it and the high is over. You miss the exercise, the people, the daily achievement.

And everything seems just ok and thus the great depression starts and unless you can shake it off some people take weeks to run again and others just days.

It's normal and we all feel it one way or another that's why we named it. It's also the reason we come back every year because those 10 days are emotionally and physically a high that you can't get from another race and the low reminds you how much you love it. Runners are always chasing that next race maybe we need to feel that running high, the achievement, have a tough goal or just have a goal that is selfishly just yours.

When I'm running nothing hurts like stopping

Charlie Harwood

Thank you, Charlie.

As challenging as this sounds, when you read words like that. You just simply must have a go. **THE GREAT BARROW CHALLENGE** http://thegbc.co.uk/

Contributors

While writing this book I reached out to several people with a request for a contribution. The running community is vast, and I was overwhelmed by the response. It seems that runners are very passionate about their sport and there was no shortage of suggestions as to what I should write about. I was sent personal stories, anecdotes, suggestions on training and nutrition and much more. Too much, in fact for one book. I want to thank everybody who has sent me information, it was brilliant. Unfortunately, as I say, far too much for one book. However, I have included as many contributions as I can, and am happy to acknowledge people by name here.

Where people have made significant contributions, these are credited within the various chapters and I have added short biographies below

Nick Jones Male age 48 (Feb 1971)

Started running in 2013 as training for Tough Mudders (first local 10k trail in 2013) as wanted to complete for charity following a relative getting Cancer, prior was boxing training (no fights), completed a few tough Mudders but thought they got a bit commercial, so started to enjoy running, met a lady in London on the day she had just finished the London Marathon (2016), she inspired me to go for ballot in 2017 and was lucky to get both a ballot and charity place (again for Cancer as uncle was dying), so took up ballot place and ran for Macmillan.

Ran up to 20 miles as part of my training, got the bug, still completed local runs including Britain's toughest 10K (Box Hill Surrey). In late 2017 my Dad got cancer so decided to do something different and got three friends (all same age roughly) together and we decided to go for Run to the Kings (53 miles along the South Downs), we followed a programme and trained up to 30 miles (3 ultra-distances as part of training). Mainly doing double day training to enhance our strength and stamina (EG: 10 miles on Sat followed by 16 miles on Sunday). It ended up being 56.7 miles!!!!

Back in 2017 was diagnosed with Asthma and take two types of inhaler, have had a cough ever since and only dec 2018 (after ultra) was diagnosed with Sarcoidosis (which is a fairly rare disease which in my case is affecting my lungs)

I was seeing a specialist while training for the ultra and they advised how 'easy' I should take it.

My times have dropped over the years and currently (2019) stand at:

10K – 48.31
50K – 6.44.58
Marathon – 3.52.43
Furthest distance: 56.7 miles in 11.59.17

Charlotte Harwood.
Marathon and ultrarunner.

Great Barrow Run Ambassador and competitor in numerous marathons and multiday endurance running events.

I have always been interested in sports psychology and playing. I played hockey until my illness made it too unsafe to play and discovered running.

I studied at DeMontfort university in Bedford. Attaining a BSc with Honours in Sports Science. I then did multiple courses in biomechanics and rehabilitation of injuries. When you do something, you love for a job it never feels like work.

When I run, I never even imagine not completing the event, it's come close a few times, but I know if I stay positive and keep going, I've done the hard work and my body just needs to keep up.

Ian Thomas Male age 60

Have been running ultramarathons for about six or so years now, I guess. I got into running seriously on the cusp of 50 but focused initially on road racing all distances from 5k to a marathon before I ventured into Ultrarunning. I've since run many ultras including the big canal races like GUCR 145 miles, Liverpool to Leeds 130 miles, the Centurion Grand Slam of 100 milers, Spartathlon 153.4 miles for the last 4 years. This year (2019)

I hope to make it 5, but you can't take anything for granted with an ultra as you know and certainly not with Spartathlon. I've also done some of Lindley Chambers events of Challenge Running and Kevin Marshall's of PositiveSteps. More recent years I've ventured into 24 hr races which present their mental challenges.

Although I've always loved running, I didn't start racing in earnest until 2009 at the age of 50, when my focus at that time was road racing everything from 5k to Marathons.

My desire is simply to be the very best that I can be and although I started a little later in life than most I guess, it's never too late to push the boundaries! Age is only a number as the saying goes!

I consider myself a competitive runner I guess but it's more about testing my limitations.

My greatest achievements include running two sub 3 marathon at Abingdon at age 52 and 53. I also completed the GUCR 145m and Thames Ring 250m at the first attempt in 2013 and have completed a total of seven of the Centurion 100 mile races in respectable times I guess, but for some reason,

I have never really excelled on the series. I improved on my GUCR time considerably in 2014 and again in 2016, finishing in 27:43 (3rd)

I was privileged to be able to run the inaugural Liverpool to Leeds 130m (LLC130) in 2014 finishing in 27:59 (8th).

I managed to improve on this in 2015 finishing in 24:09 (2nd) and although not an improved time in 2016 of 24:28, I did manage to hold on for 1st place in atrocious weather conditions.

Back in 2014 I also took on the Centurion 100-mile Grand Slam which comprised 4 x 100 mile events (The Thames Path 100, South Downs Way 100, North Downs Way 100 and the Winter 100) and was pleased to finish 6th overall in the Grand Slam table (41 started the Slam and 16 made it through.

I revisited the TP100 in 2015 and 2016 going sub 20 for the first time but have run faster 100-mile splits in longer events, hitting 17:41, 17:44, 2 x 18:00hrs, 16:47 split at my 24hr debut at Barcelona and 16:37 split at Athens 24hr in 2019.

Debuting at Spartathlon in 2015 was life-changing, but returning in 2016, 2017 and 2018 (best 29:14:36 2016), winning the Liverpool to Leeds (LLCR130) and the Essex 100 are my most recent major achievements.

Feel free to visit my blog: http://www.ultraian.wordpress.com and all the best to you with your challenges!

Ian Thomas

Glen Baddeley Male Age 48

Married, 3 kids (Two are adults now).

Age 48 3/12/70.

Been running for 28 years......though that's a bit of a lie since I stopped at around 25 until I turned 40, realized I'd put on 4 stone in weight and needed to get fit again.

I lost 3st in about 6 months.and set about training for Ironman Triathlons.

I did triathlons for about 5 years then turned my attention to Ultras.

I've done single day races in this country (35-66miles). 100miler (Robin hood 100-mile 2018). Oman Desert marathon (self-supported stage race in 2017).

I still do parkruns, and each year pick a 'non-ultra' event to try to break a significant milestone, so for example last year was to break ½ marathon 1:50, this year to break marathon 4hrs, next year 10k under 50mins....you get the idea.

About the Author

I have worked in advertising, marketing, graphic design and as a sports development consultant and disability sports coach. I've worked with BME (Black and Mixed Ethnic), mental health, homeless and people with both physical and neurological disabilities. I am a disability awareness tutor, and guest lecturer, a badminton coach, Mentor. And sometimes a creative designer. I had my own design company but decided to re-invent myself. I had always loved sport, so I became a full-time sports coach. This led to a job as a sports development officer with a local authority and developed into various consultancy positions.

Since retiring from mainstream employment in 2015, I formed a consultancy called *"Ifnotme"* which promotes equality and inclusion. It also gives me more time to follow my passion for teaching and writing. I count myself very lucky to live in a lovely part of the United Kingdom in the County of Suffolk, East Anglia with my beautiful wife Clyrene and our cat, Sam. I have a daughter, Emma and (at the time of writing, ha-ha) three gorgeous grandkids.

Also, by the author

Running with a wounded heart

The story of how I had a heart attack in my fifties during a race and recovered to run a personal best marathon time in my sixties.
Stephen Morley Copyright 2018

Mental Health in the long run

How running can improve your mental as well as your physical health.
Due for release Spring 2020

Carthorse to Racehorse

From couch potato to a thoroughbred you, one fence at a time.
Due for release September 2019.

Not your average self-help book

Are you fed up reading about *"How to Achieve Success?"*

Let me tell you about my real-life struggles and how they just might help you to live a better life
Due for release Spring 2020.

BONUS CONTENT - Podcast

A while back, I had the opportunity to record a Podcast for "CazCast" a YouTube channel run by my good friend Callum Brown. I've added a shortened transcript of the podcast here because I think it does give some context to my story. It also gives you a little background to why I wrote this second book, Too Old to Ultra. I have attempted to clean up the transcript and paraphrase where appropriate. However, it is a transcript so please forgive the duplication of some words and conversational phrases such as *"Yeah, you know"*, and the numerous *"Ers and hums"* etc.

You can find the full podcast on YouTube: https;//www.youtube.com/watch?v=YOYOu7 ZZHBI

CazCast. Published on Feb 7, 2019

"Today's episode is nothing short of incredible with author Steve Morley. When running a 7-mile race Steve had a heart attack, in this Podcast Steve talks about what happened that day and tells us about the years after and how he has found a love for running ultra-marathons.

After a short introduction, I was asked to read a short extract from my book, Running with a wounded heart. I read the preface which told the story of me experiencing what I later realized was a heart attack.

Callum: "Wow, that is gripping. Just listening to you saying that now and just reliving it, you know you feel like you understand the emotions of it and yeah, I can't imagine how you felt in that moment. As someone that does a lot of training and exercise myself, there are times when I'm training, when I am pushing really hard but I know my body so well that I know the difference between being uncomfortable because you're pushing yourself to your limits and perhaps you know something is just not right with your body. For you, that must have been a unique feeling at the time. Did you think at all that you were having a heart attack?"

Steve: "No, not at all. There's a famous story. Do you know the comedy duo, Morecambe and Wise? Well Eric Morecambe, bless him, he had lots of heart problems and ultimately it killed him. He told a very funny story about the first time he had a heart attack. He said he was out driving somewhere, and he felt unwell and he said he saw a policeman directing traffic. He was somewhere, in an area he wasn't familiar with and he pulled over asked the policeman to tell him where the nearest hospital was. So the policeman directed him to the hospital and the interviewer said to him, exactly what you just asked me - so did you know you were having a heart attack and he said, not at all, he said if I'd have thought I was having a heart attack I'd have had a heart attack. So, to answer your question, no I didn't know I was having a heart attack.

I honestly didn't know what it was. People often say, when you have a heart attack or a bad case of angina or any of those kinds of symptoms, where there's a blockage in your heart that it feels much like intense indigestion.

The thing is, I've always been a fit guy and, it sounds strange but, I can't ever remember ever having indigestion. I always eat well, and I eat properly.

I'm not one of these people that rush about with a sandwich in one hand and a can of drink or a coffee in the other, running from A to B and so I've never been in a situation where I've given myself indigestion or I've had heartburn or anything like that. So, I've never had any of those situations where I could recognize the symptoms.

So, I couldn't compare it. However, in my head, I was thinking if I had had indigestion maybe this is what it would feel like, okay that kind of feeling".

(reading the chapter of the book that tells the story of my admission to and stay at the hospital)

Callum: "Wow, yeah how does that make you feel now, just like reading that back. How do you feel about that situation and since that happened, I mean, how has that changed you would you say?"

Steve: "Well quite a lot of water has gone under the bridge since then. That was 2010 and we're nine years on now.

I occasionally I read it to people and I feel a bit emotional when I'm reading it but the good thing about what happened was that in the year that it took me to recover I started running again and I promised myself I was going to run the race again.

Everybody said, yeah, I had nothing to prove I shouldn't run the race again. Well, I was determined to kind of get back on the horse and I describe it in the book as slaying the dragon. I think it's important you know, I got trashed by the dragon, even got carted off to the hospital. So, it was important but the funny thing about it was. my friend Kevin and my friend Lee, both ran with me during the race. I told them that I wanted to run my race and they said, oh yeah sure, we will let you run your race but, you know they were never too far away.

They were always keeping an eye on me during the race. Here's the funny thing. I got to the hill where I had the heart attack and I wondered how I would feel running up the hill and passing the spot. So, I'm running up the hill and I'm trying to remember the exact point where I had the heart attack. I'm thinking, I think it was here, no, no, It, wasn't here it was a bit further up. Was it here? No, it wasn't but, and then I got to the top of the hill and realized you know what? yeah, I must have passed it and I couldn't remember where it was.

So, going up the hill that was funny, that made me laugh out loud and then I finished the race and burst into tears which was a bit wimpy of me and Kevin and Lee were also like, you know, like guys are not very good with that sort of thing.

However, I knew that they were looking up at the heaven and whistling. That was the only bit of emotion."

Callum: "Sure, yeah because, you know, when you were running, you're being strong, but it must have always been there in the back of your mind a little bit and leading up to that race. I mean how long was that? How long apart was that from when the time it happened to you running the race again?

Steve: "The next year."

Callum: "So it was, the next year. So, it was exactly a year yes so yeah. I mean I think that's incredible.

When that happened, you know, the day after that happened did you ever think that you would be running back in that same race the following year?"

Steve: "Yes, I was determined to do that yeah. When I was in the hospital. I got taken in on a Sunday and on the Monday morning the doctor came and did his rounds. It was the first question I asked him. I said to him, when can I expect to be running again?

(reading the chapter of the book that tells the continues the story from the hospital)

Callum: "Thank you very much, Stephen, for reading that because that is, you know, that's a hell of a thing for anyone to go through.

So, you know the fact that you've now written a book about it to help other people and you've come on here to speak about it I think it's amazing. I think people are going to take a lot from those extracts there so yeah, I can't thank you enough for that. So, what I'd like to do now is move on to your second book which you have coming out which is called Too old to ultra. So, let's just start by giving the listeners a bit of information about what that book is okay?"

Steve: Well when I recovered from my heart attack, I started running again and it took me I suppose it took me a year probably maybe just over a year to feel that I was fully recovered and shortly after that I ran my first post-heart attack marathon. If memory serves me it was Luton, the Luton marathon which is a horrible marathon.

I have to say that. Apologies to anybody who's running or has run that marathon, but it's a horrible marathon. it's like in December, it's cold and it's got lots of hills in it. Yes, it's not a lot of fun, not one of my favorites. My favorite marathon is probably Milton Keynes because it's nice and flat, yeah and it finishes in the football stadium which is great so as you run around the running track you see yourself on the big screen so that's good. But yeah so, I got back, and I'd ran a couple of marathons and that was good. I was okay doing that and but I kind of...... I'm always looking to improve and one of the things that often happens when you get older is you can improve but you must change the parameters a little bit. So, where running is concerned, you know, forget about trying to improve your 5k time.

Forget about trying to improve your 10k time, because your fast twitch muscles are not there anymore and it's not going to happen no matter how hard you try.

Well, it is going to happen, but it is going to be incrementally. You are probably not going to knock big chunks off your 5k time in your sixties, it's just not going to happen yeah? However, the longer distances you run, the more room for improvement there is. So, you start off doing a five-hour marathon and you do training and you work hard, you can do a four-hour marathon and if you push harder and you push on to and train, you can do it like a three and a half hour marathon you know?

With ultra-running, it's a kind of whole different ballgame. So, you're running much longer distances. The whole thing is kind of different from a marathon in all sorts of ways.

So, in a marathon, 26 miles 26 and bit miles, you have stations, food stations and invariably they'll have paper cups of water or they might have isotonic drinks, so they might have jelly babies or something like that. In an ultra-marathon, it's like a running buffet so it's like pretzels and crisps and peanuts whatever you need just get calories in because you want the salt, yeah and they need the protein. So, it's a whole different ballgame and the marshaling is different because you know in a marathon you've got marshals everywhere, every mile or so and at junctions and such.

In an ultra-marathon, they are few and far between and you must rely on running notes. So, it's a whole different challenge and I got just intrigued by the idea of it. I said, well I can run 26 miles can I run 30 miles? because technically speaking anything over 32 miles is classified as an ultra over 32 yeah?

Callum: "So what about anything in between 26 for 32?"

Steve: "It's like, its people's perception of it yeah? If you run, a lot of people say, well I did I think King's forest. That is 30 miles that's around where the Saxon villages yep it's just a nice round number to label really yeah and you know they qualify that as an ultra.

So, yeah, depends how strict you want to be but yeah if you read up on it you know, sort of marathon distance is 26.2 or 4 whereas 30 to 32 miles and above qualifies as an ultra. So, you get a lot of what I call baby ultras which are like 30 to 35 miles. Peddars way, which was the first one I attempted that's 47 I think or nearly 48 miles. Yeah, so a lot of them that are about that sort of distance. I did a couple of the shorter ones to see if I could do it and then I attempted Peddars as my first adventure or as it turned out my misadventure.

(reading the first chapter of the book, Too Old to Ultra. That and some other sample chapters are included in this book.)

Callum: Doesn't sound ideal for your first ultra-marathon. Not a good start (laughs).

So, how long was this race?

Steve: 47/48 miles.

Callum: And when did this happen.

Steve: 18 miles.

Callum: 18 miles, wow. So, it was all going well till then?

Steve: Yes, I'd settled into my run. I was feeling ok. I had recced the route over the previous weeks. So, what we used to do was break the route down into small sections. It's what I still do. Break the route down into small sections and then every week I'd go with a friend and he would drop me off.

He would then drive maybe 20 miles to an agreed point. I'd then run that 20 miles section of the ultra. We would then come back the next week and do a different section of the route. So, for weeks, you are using your training runs to become familiar with the route.

But the thing about Peddars, because of the time of year, it gets dark. So, you are running the final stages of the race with only a head torch to see where you are going. So, whereas everything looks fine and dandy in the daytime, everything looks completely different in the dark.

Callum: I can imagine, you know, that it gives you like a bit of an edge knowing you've run this before even though it's not the entire run but knowing that you've actually hit this section before and you know that can also give you an idea of time and pacing. So, when you're looking at running that 47 miles did you have a goal in terms of time and how did you work out what pace you needed to go for that race?"

Steve: Well, apart from a couple of baby ultras. that was my first proper one. So, I just wanted to finish it, yeah and it's a strange thing about ultramarathons in as much as in many ways they're very generous.

They seem very daunting but they're very generous with respect to the amount of time they give you to complete it. So, in the case of peddars, I think the official cut off time is about 12 hours

If you do the math you could probably almost walk it in that time you know. Stepping out you could almost walk it. So, if you can run a bit and walk when you need to, run a bit and walk a bit, you can kind of do it providing you prepare for it. I intended to finish it but, here's the thing about that first ultra. I probably shouldn't have run it because the weather conditions were bad and leading up to the race it was heavy snow and cold. In the days leading up to the race, they kept posting on social media stay tuned we may have to cancel and lots of people dropped out lots of people said, this is ridiculous,

I'm not doing this. So, when we got there on the day out of about 250 people that had put their names down to enter there was only about 120 people turned up. So, a whole lot of people had dropped out and even then, it was like what should we do? The organizers are in a little huddle and in the end, they did the worst possible thing they could do, they asked us.

So, of course, they're saying who'd like to carry on and of course, nobody wants to like put their hands in their pockets. Everyone said they've turned up ready to go so yeah, we all put our hands up.

What they should have done is taken responsibility and said like I'm sorry guys we've had to talk about this we've had to look at the weather that's coming your way.

The weather accounts look bad and sorry but for safety, we are going to have to cancel. Instead, they said what do you guys want to do? So, we all set off and snow got heavier and heavier I'd got to 18 miles I'd got to go from 18 miles to 23 miles hobbling. I got lost several times because the snow had covered all the markers over. As I said before, there were no marshals about. The funniest thing, and not being overly critical of the organizers, but when I told people I was going to it (run Peddars) they said Oh, what about your safety and I said well they must look after you mustn't they? Probably what they do, maybe you'll get an electronic chip or something so maybe they'll be able to monitor you. See where you are. You know, you've fallen down this drainage ditch and somebody notices.

Oh, hang on, number 604 hasn't moved for the last 20 minutes, (laughs) maybe we should send somebody to see if they are okay. Yeah, and one of the elite runners maybe they come back. yes, or send someone on a mountain bike, or something, come and look for you. No, forget it, none of that.

The funniest thing was when I got to the halfway part, all I was thinking was, there'll be a nice welcoming checkpoint with friendly marshals with hot soup and coffee and food and everything you know. When I got to the halfway, what? they'd packed it all away. It had all been packed up and not a buttered toll in sight. Fortunately, there was a pub nearby and I made my way to the pub and the people that had been marshaling at the halfway point we're in the pub having their lunch.

When I came through the door covered in snow and with freezing blue lips, one of the ladies, in between eating her lunch, she stopped, picked up a mobile phone and she said hello control, number 604 has just come in - how many is it now we're missing? Apparently, seven people got hypothermia, a whole load of people dropped out and they had brought the cut-off point forward because the weather had got so bad. So, I couldn't have continued at that point even if I'd have wanted to because they were not letting any more runners come through.

Callum: Since doing your ultra, do now realize that okay this one just wasn't run well or is there a common factor with ultras that you are always going to a little bit vulnerable?

Steve: I think you are encouraged to be self-reliant right and you need to be self-reliant so it's really important to have a team it's not like I mean, I've done marathons before I've just taken myself off on my own and run them parked the car, I run the marathon driven home again. For something like an ultra, you need a support team so you know like you need a good friend or you know like my brother-in-law or somebody like that who you plan it out so that they're at a lay-by on the side of the A1 or wherever.

You need that extra support. At one of the ultras, I think it might have Peddars again, there were two people a young woman and a man, both evenly matched. One finished and one didn't, and the last checkpoint is about 13 miles before the finish and when I did it in the recce I said to the person I was running with, if I can get here I'll finish it because I know I'm not going to let the last 13 miles beat me. If I can get here, I'll crawl the last 13 miles if I must.

The boy didn't finish it and the girl did and the difference was the boy got there was nobody to help him. He had a coffee, hot coffee, set off ran 400 yards turned around and walked back and rang up and said come and get me I can't do it I just come to get me.

The girl had her husband or partner I can't remember in a car she had a hot coffee she took a hot coffee into the car right lovely warm car she changed her shoes but nice clean warm socks on he took off her top put a new warm top on got her gloves off put nice warm gloves on and she sat there for 20 minutes getting warmed up yeah before getting out of the car then going again nailing the last 13 miles. Yep and that was the difference just having that a little bit of support.

Callum: I imagine for some people having that comfort and that warmth would have made it even harder to get back out there. It depends on your personality, I guess.

Steve: There is a famous ultra that goes along like the length of Hadrian's Wall and that's like an all-nighter yeah and a friend, I have not run it, but a friend of mine who ran it said a van comes along in the middle of the night, early hours of the morning, a van comes along and stops and they opened the doors and you get in and you can have hot coffee and things yeah, and get warm and he said, you know, I got in and you know they drive along a little bit further you know, pick up the next group and he's sitting there and then the driver said, well I can't keep driving you down your road. You are going to have to get or stay yeah? and he said they open the doors he had that shall I go or shall I moment. He said, yeah, I was like every fibre of my body just wanted to stay in the warm.

He said it took all my willpower to get out of the car. Ironically, he said, once I was out within a few minutes of being out I was alright again it's just that little moment of respite that gives you the strength to carry on.

Callum: So, let's pick it up from where you go down that ditch, yeah and you said about you had to hobble along, I mean had you injured yourself what happened to you after that?

Steve: yeah it was I was lucky I was at the bottom of the ditch and I was staring up like and snowflakes were falling on my face, gently falling on my face yeah? Everything was quiet and still.

You couldn't hear anything and then I kind of had to think, right now have I hurt myself is anything broken yeah? and I kind of I sort of moved my fingers and moved my toes and everything moves everything seemed to work okay so I kind of got myself sitting up and then I had to retrieve all my stuff. My water bottle had gone one way and another drinks bottle had gone another way and things had come out of my utility belt. I had my utility belt stuffed with Mars bars and yeah and energy bars and energy gels and things and they'd all gone everywhere.

So, I had to collect all these things and then clamber up the side of this ditch and about halfway up I realize my foot was sore. I'd obviously hurt my foot or ankle so I started to run but it was too painful to run right so I knew I couldn't go on.

I knew I sprained it or strained it or something and I had nothing to strap it up with yeah and so I persevered but I kind of knew at that point I was probably not going to be able to finish. I had a mobile phone with me and rang my son-in-law and said, I need you to come to Castle Acre. I'm going to try and get to Castle Acre and can you come and pick me from up there. Which is what he did.

I was very disappointed in the fact that I wasn't going to be able to finish – but the things that were sustaining me one was I knew that Rob was on his way to pick me up, so I knew I was getting collected. That was fine, someone's coming to get me, and the second thing was the thought of having like this nice hot soup - you know - kind of re-energize me.

And, you know what yeah? what was so disappointing was that when I arrived, there was nothing there, it had all been packed away.

So, that was the hardest thing. Fortunately, the pub was open, so that made things a little bit better. Yeah, I didn't have any beer I just got a big mug of coffee perfect just to warm me up.

Callum: So, one thing that I wanted to ask you about Stephen was the physical effects. If we start with that the physical effects of doing ultramarathons on the body. The positive effects in terms of, you know cardiovascular benefits and you know how incredibly fit you can get an increase in your endurance but also is there a detrimental effect on the body in terms of longevity?

When you complete in these ultra-marathons and you know, what is the sort of the science behind that or what do you know about it?

Steve: Well the jury is out when it comes to long-distance running. I think most people in the medical profession would agree that exercise is good for you I don't think you have any question on that and I think most people would say that running is good for you when you

are doing a lot of running. whether that's a lot of heavy training or

whether you're running long distances, then you've got to think about just the physical stress on your joints for a start.

I was talking to somebody at the gym recently who was about to do a marathon and was so disappointed because they'd started getting knee problems. When I spoke to them about it, it was the fact that they'd been doing all their training on the pavement, you know on the roads. I'm lucky where I live because I can run around the warren in Lakenheath so when Ie and I do our long runs, we do laps of the Warren*. You have the benefit that it was nice and soft underfoot, so you weren't put too much strain on your joints but because it was undulating, it was helping your core strength and balance. and so, it was good in that respect but doing long distances, well there are a lot of studies that say maybe it's not good for you.

I always like to compare running an ultra to running a marathon and I maintain that running an ultra is not as detrimental to your health potentially as running a marathon.

When you run a marathon, I mean, when you get to the point where you're running a four-hour marathon, three and a half, three-hour marathons, you know you are doing ten-minute nine minutes eight-minute milling and most marathons are run on the road. So, for 26 miles even if you're only running at like eight-minute mile pace you're putting quite a big strain on your body and your heart. If you run an ultra, you're not running an eight-minute mile pace you know you're running at maybe you're running a ten-minute mile pace, 11 minutes, 12-minute miles plus.

So, although you're running farther, you're not running as fast and, unless you're an elite ultra-runner, you're often walking quite a lot at the time as well, so your heart rate comes down because you're walking. You can recover a bit and you go again. So, overall, even though you're running a lot longer, you're not placing as big a strain on your body as you would in a marathon.

Callum: I know what you mean. It's almost more natural to the body in terms of, that it involves walking and you know you are dependent on the route you're doing you might have to go up some hills it's flat. It can be, it's a very varied experience for your body.

There are some intense moments in there where you are going to be maxing your heart rate up, but you are going to be bringing things back down and it's more of a longevity thing.

It was interesting, I have listened to a podcast recently and there's a guy called Ross Edgeley who swam around the UK and if you look at him he looks like a powerlifter, very muscular very broad he's like he looks really heavy and the guy who was interviewing him said don't take offense to this but you don't look like a swimmer. I'm very surprised that your body shape looks like this and you've swum around the UK.

I was expecting someone to be sort of tall lean athletic more athletic but the way he described it was like he was imagining, and he pictured himself like a whale. Yes, just going around the UK but at a very slow pace but just very consistent and being very durable and obviously having extreme like mental strength because most of the time his head was in the water and he was just amongst his thoughts it's going to be really tough and so that's what I'd like to go onto now, the mental side of running an ultra-marathon which is equally as challenging as getting in physical shape, I imagine. So, in terms of when you're training for a marathon in terms of mentally preparation, are you doing anything to help and improve your mental strength?

Is that something that you've always found easy do you keep your mind clear, or do you think about things to make the time go faster? What's your approach with that?

Steve: Ok, so one of the training things that I do, is bizarre really because it doesn't involve any running at all. One of the things that I do at least once or twice when I'm training for an ultra is, I'd go out all day and I'm on my feet the whole day.

So, I pick myself a route that, ideally is a big loop, it's maybe 20-plus miles, you know, in a loop and the only time I jog is to relieve the boredom. Mostly I just walk so I'm just walking and I'm out all day.

So, I might leave home at 8 am with the intention that I won't be back, it will take me all day to get back home again yeah and because it's a loop I must do it. So, there is no point doing small loops because you set out to do eight loops and after you've done four or five, you think, to hell with this, that will do for today, you know, because you're coming past your house again and you think, do I really want to go around again. If you do a big loop you get to the point of no return where it's going to take you longer to turn around and go back, okay, so you might as well just keep going because you've got to get home back home right? You can't stay out there.

That's usually the only the time in the run that I do run. To relieve the boredom and to hurry up and get home. However, just being on your feet all day, yeah that is good

mental training knowing if you can do that.

But, yes for sure, the mental side of it is very hard because often it's very lonely. Unless you find yourself running with a group of other runners, it is quite lonely. One of the first runs I did, I got quite friendly with a girl on Facebook. She was doing the same ultra and we exchanged ideas. I made the fatal mistake of asking her if she fancied running it together and we support one another.

She was very polite and diplomatic, but she said no, and she explained why, and she said. Because you get into this head place where if you're struggling and somebody's saying now come on, we can do this together, it gets irritating and I mean you can get aggressive and angry when you are cold and tired.

When you feel that your partner is struggling you feel like you've got to

slow down and support them and it messes your head up and yeah. She said too many potential emotional ups and downs, yeah. She said that, you know, if we find that we happen to be running together and we're having a little chat then fine but let's not do it as a plan yeah because you know if you or your partner have to drop out, yeah and It's like, you feel, maybe I've got to drop out as well yeah okay.

No, you say, we'll go back together you know don't worry you know it just messes with your brain. So, she said to me you must do it on your own you can't do it with a buddy So all the ones I've done, I've done on my own. I try to get Mr. Le to come with me and he just thinks I'm crazy

Many thanks to Callum Brown and CazCast

You can listen to the full podcast on YouTube: https;//www.youtube.com/watch?v=YOYOu7 ZZHBI

Thank you and final thoughts

I write these books for people like me; people, who are not in the first flush of youth, people who perhaps are beginners or low-level runners. People who maybe have had heart-related issues or whose health is not great; people who aspire to run but because of their age or health feel they just can't. Maybe that's true, maybe it's not. Until you try you don't know. My wife has a great saying;

"If you can't ride a horse, ride a cow"

So, if you can't run then jog and if you can't jog then walk.

And, if you can't walk, well – sitting outside with the sun on your face isn't so bad.

"The answers to the big questions in running are the same as the answers to the big questions in life: Do the best with what you've got. And, sometimes you may find that you have GOT more than you think."

Thank you for taking the time out to read my book. I hope that you enjoyed it.

You can follow me on Social Media. My Author Facebook page is to be found at: https://www.facebook.com/wriitenbyme/
If you liked the book, I would appreciate it if you can leave a review on Amazon.

Good luck with your running and thanks again.

Steve